The

Kaufmann

Protocol

Legal Notice and Disclaimer

The information provided in this book is based upon peer-reviewed and published medical studies. Dr. Kaufmann's analyses and conclusions based on these studies are, however, for informational purposes only and are not meant to replace the guidance and advice of your licensed physician or other healthcare practitioners. Statements in this book have not been evaluated by the Food and Drug Administration for, inter alia, drug interactions, warnings, or alerts.

The information provided is meant for general use only and is not intended to diagnose, cure, treat, or prevent any diseases or conditions, or to provide medical advice. Any decision to use the supplements and medicines discussed should be considered in partnership with your licensed physician or other healthcare practitioner.

Cover design by Ross Goldstein
Book design and production by Amy Steinberg

The Kaufmann Protocol
Copyright © 2017 Sandra Kaufmann, MD

The Kaufmann Protocol

WHY WE AGE
AND HOW TO STOP IT

WRITTEN BY
SANDRA KAUFMANN, MD

EDITED BY
JACOB CERNY

ILLUSTRATIONS BY
ROSS GOLDSTEIN

Dedicated to all the mice and rats that have given up
their lives to help the rest of us live better and longer.

PERSONAL STATEMENT

I am a physician, a scientist, a mother, and an athlete. But most importantly, I am a woman who decided a few years ago that I loved my life, and didn't want it destroyed by the seemingly inevitable thing we call aging. So, rather than give in with grace, I decided to fight... with grace.

The biggest weapons I had in my arsenal were my background, my brain and my determination, so the battle began.

To start, I am a scientist by training. As an undergrad, I discovered a dispersal mechanism for an invasive plant species which prompted me to pursue a Masters Degree in Ecology and Evolutionary Biology with an emphasis on cellular plasticity under changing environmental conditions. I spent years studying cells and coming to understand their intricacies.

I then invested over a decade learning human physiology, biology and pharmacology in Medical School and Residency, completing my fellowship at Johns Hopkins. At present, I am the Chief of Pediatric Anesthesia at the Joe DiMaggio Children's Hospital in Florida. I am also an athlete. I hang from cliffs and I climb mountains. I swim, I run, I bike. I, of all people, understand exercise physiology.

People ask, why me? The answer is simple.

I know cells, I know research, I know the human body. I was determined. And now, I know how to stop aging.

F O R W A R D

There are several items that need to be addressed prior to reading this book.

Most importantly, when people talk about anti-aging, the first thing that comes to mind is 'bullshit.' I don't doubt that most folks reading this have a very low threshold for thinking this is all quite ridiculous. In fact, I assumed the same thing years ago as various reports of miracle anti-aging agents would pop into and out of the news. That is until, one day in my 40's, I had had it with aging. I was perfectly content where I was, but I was not willing to fall down the seemingly inevitable downward spiral. I didn't want to look old, I didn't want to feel old, and I certainly didn't want to act old. In what has been called the most productive outcome of a mid-life crisis, I set out to overcome aging… but in a logical way. I began plowing through thousands and thousands of legitimate, scientific research papers to determine if there was anything of substance I could do to stave off the effects of time.

To my gleeful shock, I was thrilled to discover that there was an entire world of science and research that was already battling this challenge and making real, actual strides. Therefore, everything that is presented in this book comes directly from real science - from brilliant researchers in renown universities, around the globe, uncovering real solutions. You will find no citations from Men's Health, Women's Day magazine nor any opinions from pseudo experts on television. Every bit of information comes from the source.

Unfortunately, as I have discovered, these sources are a little dry in the entertainment department. If you care to browse the actual articles, I have included all of the references; you can try reading them at your leisure. Therefore, I decided that my job was two fold. First, I have translated the scientific information into understandable concepts. It really isn't fair that the only people who are aware of these anti-aging strategies aren't sharing them with the rest of the nonscientific world. In fact, it took me years to weed through all of the information and turn it into a cohesive doctrine. After all that time, it seemed a little selfish to keep the information all to myself.

Secondly, I hope to entertain you as well.

It is also important to note that this is NOT a book about diet and exercise. This is not a weight loss program; it is not a fad, nor is it a gimmick. There is no 30 day trial, no mention of carbohydrates and no ketones. There are no references to what the paleolithic people consumed, nor any colon cleansing. This is about aging, and aging ONLY. In fact, the focus of this book is cellular health. It is a given that a good diet and exercise can be beneficial to health, so we are going far, far beyond this.

Another important aspect to consider is that understanding this topic, by default, will encompass very scientific information. As with any difficult topic, it contains innumerable levels of complexity, and it is my responsibility to determine where a reasonable threshold lies; and as everyone reading this will have varying degrees of scientific background to begin with, no one will be completely happy with its presentation. For some, the details will seem overwhelming and unnecessary. For others, my information will seem superficial and leave them craving additional knowledge.

All things being said, have a little patience. Enjoy the read, live a little longer and have a better life.

The **K** aufmann

P rotocol

CHAPTER 1

INTRODUCTION

Aging is much like beauty. It is easy to recognize, but incredibly difficult to explain or understand. We can see aging in people around us; we notice changes in facial structure, fat deposition, energy levels and even enthusiasm for life. We can feel age in ourselves. We look in the mirror and see hairs where they shouldn't be, and the lack of hair where we need it. We see greater folds of skin around our nose and looser skin over our eyes. Perhaps we notice our vision slipping; night vision not quite as crisp, and then there is the dreaded need to borrow reading glasses in a dark restaurant.

Even worse, we all know what the beginning of aging feels like. The first time, somewhere around the mid-thirties, you realize that you are not immortal. This realization can be ugly. Until that time, life was effortless: injuries healed quickly, skin was beautiful (with the exception of acne in the teenage years), it was easy to remain slim, you could consume pretty much whatever you wanted and could stay up all night without ramifications. However, somewhere in the third decade, things start to change. At this point, we are no longer on the upswing; we are either leveling off or just starting the decline. Everyone of us is on this spectrum somewhere, and even if we don't talk about it, everyone has to deal with it in their own way.

Despite the universality of this phenomena, scientists still struggle with a definition of aging. It has been described as many things, none of which sound very appealing:

> *"Aging is associated with a generalized decline in all physiological functions, and between 30 and 70 we are likely to observe a 25-30% reduction on most functional capacities."*[1]

> *"A deterioration in the maintenance of homeostatic processes over time leading to functional decline and increased risk of death and disease..."*[2]

> *"Aging is a complex multifactorial process of molecular and cellular decline that affects tissue function over time, rendering organisms frail and susceptible to disease and death."*[3]

So, the best place to start this quest is to state the obvious: we all are going to get old and die. It's a bit depressing, but unfortunately accurate. Traditionally, the only other option is to die prematurely, which isn't enviable either. Despite this self-evident truth, over the millennia, the conditions under which we age have changed dramatically. Thousands of years ago, the average lifespan was about 30 years. It was just enough time to grow up, have a few children and then croak.

There were notable exceptions, of course. Ramses the Great, for example, was 90 years old when he died in 1213 BC. It's good to be the king.

Funny helps too! George Burns and Bob Hope both lived to 100

In the never-ending battle to curtail aging, very enthusiastic people have tried very creative methods for avoiding the inevitable. The fabled fountain of youth was described by Herodotus in the 5th century BC, in a land belonging to the Macrobians.

They do have quite the population of old people

Very old sources also place the fountain in India, Bimini and most recently, St. Augustine, Florida.

The idea of imbibing an elixir to obtain everlasting life is transcultural. Amrit, the nectar of immortality, was popularized in the Hindu scriptures in India. Consumption of gold and mercury was thought to confer immortality in ancient China. Qin Shi Huang, the infamous first emperor of China, builder of the Great Wall and the buried terra cotta warriors, was obsessed with immortality. Unfortunately, in his quest, he perished of mercury poisoning at the age of 49. Clearly, nothing has worked quite yet.

Despite the ultimate failure of these attempts, the average lifespan, as well as the quality of life or health span, is in fact higher than it has ever been.

The average length of life, until fairly recently, was rather low. In 1900, the mean anticipated age was only 47. This factors in the high rate of child mortality, so it isn't completely representative. Regardless, by 2010, it had risen to 77. In Japan today, it is 83.7. Here in the U.S., we are sitting at 79.3.

Improvements in living conditions, work environments, sanitation, food preparation, and medical therapies have helped significantly. Childhood mortality has declined, and death during childbirth has also been dramatically reduced in the developed world. People are now living well into their eighties and nineties regularly, while the number of centenarians has reached record numbers. The number of supercentenarians, those over the age of 110, has also increased to an estimated 400 folks world wide. Of note, one in a thousand centenarians get to be supercentenarians.

Presently, the oldest living person in the world is 115, but the record remains at 122.5 years. In the U.S. in 2010, there were 53,000 people over the age of 100, of which 82% were women, and presently there are 40 people over the age of 110.

Lifespan and health span are now considered by some to be pushed to the upper limits of the human condition. Therefore, given a healthy diet, appropriate exercise, good genes and an abundance of fortunate circumstances, they cap us off at about 115.

It has become clear, however, at least in the scientific literature, that we haven't actually reached the ceiling. Scientists and physicians, and everyone really, have traditionally considered aging and physiological changes with aging as inevitable. Fortunately, this view has slowly eroded as we untangle the actual mechanisms of aging.

If we can understand WHY we age, it may be very possible to curtail this process. Realizing this sounds a bit quixotic, we are sitting in a very unique position in time and space. Communication between cultures has never been greater, and thus healing traditions and secrets are now not only readily available to all, but they can be studied.

As well, scientific knowledge and equipment is beyond amazing. Not only can we sequence DNA, but quantify specific errors in the DNA. We can even measure DNA destruction rates and incredibly small aliquots of enzymes. We can follow specific genes as they get transcribed and processed and peer into the smallest corners of our cells to reveal their secrets.

Equally as important, computers have made this information available to anyone. For example, scientists in Japan are studying microscopic cellular changes after treatment with ancient Indian herbs, mixed with Hawaiian algae, and I can read all about it in my living room in Miami.

With all this in mind, the first step to approaching this project of anti-aging is to answer the obvious question - Why do we age at all?

This has been debated for years and the answer is clearly not a simple one. We are complicated beings with innumerable levels of intrinsic complexity and interrelated systems that can deviate in any of a number of places. There are, however, very specific theories that have evolved over the last two decades.

The good news is that not only are there theories of aging, but there are also substantiated ways to block, or at least slow down, the process. A select set of scientists appear to be aware of this, but it seems that no one else does. In fact, it took me years to uncover all of the relevant information, synthesize it

If you already do, please proceed to second half of the book now

Having curtailed my own aging, I had plenty of time on my hands

and figure out what was applicable in the real world. So, I could just tell you what to do, but would you believe me?

Therefore, in order to disseminate this information and educate anyone who wants to know, I have spent an inordinate amount of time organizing these ideas into a cohesive model, which is outlined in the next chapter.

PART 1

CHAPTER 2:

THE BODY AS A FACTORY

The human body is a large and complex factory. It is not a simple, linear Henry Ford assembly line, but a complex, sophisticated system composed of innumerable, criss-crossing and circular pathways that must conform in time and space. We may, in fact, be the most complicated factory that has ever existed.

Regardless, we still function as a standard factory and thus have the same requirements. Therefore, to understand the body, we need to understand a factory. Independent of whether or not you've actually set foot in a factory, this is going to be a simple analogy; lengthy, but simple. Let's start with the basics. In order to get our factory running, we are going to consider all of the obvious aspects, such as an operating manual, a maintenance department, security, employees…you get the picture.

So, without further ado, the human body as played by a factory.

The first thing a factory needs is the written word; the standard operating or instruction manual. That is, exactly WHAT the factory is going to produce, and HOW is it going to accomplish this goal. If this was a car manufacturing plant, for example, we first would decide on the type of automobile to be produced, such as a convertible or an SUV. We then need to know specifics - frame size, the color of the seats, the type of engine; the list of details is enormous. Lastly, we would follow the step by step guide as to how to actually make the darn thing.

Our human factory needs similar instructions and details, and all of this resides in our DNA. The nature and structure of DNA will be addressed elsewhere, but it is important to note that every instruction in the body is inscribed in, and dictated by, the DNA.

By every instruction, I literally mean every instruction! Like anything produced in a factory, we need instructions for the big stuff, like being a human in the first place and the number of fingers on each hand, but we also need the blueprints for the most specific of details, like eye color and hair texture.

We actually carry instructions for every protein, fiber, cell and enzyme within our DNA. The amount of information that our DNA carries is almost unfathomable, but remarkably, the system works.

Usually!

The next thing every factory requires is energy. Nothing functions without energy, especially the human body. Some factories rely on the electrical grid, while some produce their own energy via coal, hydroelectric, or even nuclear sources. Regardless, fuel, of some nature, is imported and then altered to provide the necessary power. The body, of course, has much the same system. We import energy in the form of food and consequently calories, and then convert it into usable energy. Once in the body, the food gets broken down into smaller and smaller chunks and eventually, once at the molecular level, it gets transported into organelles called mitochondria. Here, the chemical energy gets converted into the currency of the body, a molecule called ATP. Don't panic, however, mitochondria and organelles will be explained later, in quite a bit of detail. You will soon know all about how your body is giving you the energy to read this book.

Medical Prefixes 101 ▶

A molecule of adenosine with one attached phosphate is called adenosine <u>mono</u>phosphate. If you add a second, it becomes <u>di</u>phosphate. Three, therefore is adenosine <u>tri</u>phosphate.

It takes energy to glue the phosphates together, and this energy becomes harnessed and stored within the bonds. When required, a phosphate can be removed and the energy is consequently released. The constant shuffling of phosphates provides the energy for every reaction that is required within the body.

We now have the written instructions and an energy system for our factory; the next requirement includes the work flows or predetermined pathways. Composed of assembly lines, supply chains, feedback loops, and control systems, these are necessary so that the system flows efficiently.

In the body, there are countless numbers of these pathways. There are hormonal pathways that control a balance of progesterone and estrogen for egg production. There are feedback loops for bone maintenance, and calcium and phosphate balance. There are feedback loops in kidneys to determine how concentrated or dilute urine should be, and in the brainstem telling you when and how deeply to breath.

In essence, they are everywhere.

In terms of aging, we are going to focus on energy pathways as these seem to be most relevant. Therefore, we are going to consider the sirtuin pathway, the AMP Kinase pathway and then the mTOR system. I am mentioning these briefly here, but you will hear plenty more about them shortly.

There are actually several more age-related pathways and feedback loops we could discuss, but for now, these should suffice.

In short, depending on the organismal or the cellular nutritional status, these pathways are either activated or deactivated, and serve to control energy allotment and growth. In times of deprivation or caloric restriction, growth and catabolism are limited and the body becomes more conservative with its energy. Of note, this metabolic slowdown is associated with an increasing lifespan in almost all organisms studied. Thus, these pathways are quite important to us.

Continuing the factory analogy, we come to the department of Quality Control. When a factory is small, say only a few employees and a single product; quality control is easy. It is not challenging to spot a substandard job done by a lackadaisical employee. In a huge system, however, frequent checks and quality assessments must be done at every level to ensure the steady production of a perfect product. The body, of course, is the same. Every protein that is produced is checked and double checked by "inspector proteins."

They have hard hats and clipboards too!

Likewise, DNA is constantly monitored for wear and tear. As the system ages, i.e., the factory gets older, an ever-increasing number of things go wrong: protein production fails, DNA gets compromised, organelles malfunction, etc. Therefore, the cellular quality control and repair mechanisms continuously expand their duties over time in order to maintain a functional system.

The security system is also an integral part of the complex. Instead of security cameras, high electrical fences and overweight security guards, the body has its own complex system. Our skin serves as the outer defense system, while internally we have an extensive immunologic system consisting of a roaming force of trouble spotting cells. These cells, phagocytes, macrophages, T cells, B cells, eosinophils, basophils, mast cells and my favorite, the natural killer cells, travel around the body eradicating anything that looks troublesome.

It's your body's own Department of Homeland Security

This system functions fairly well when we are young, but unfortunately, many of these cells go rogue with time, turning a benevolent system into a malicious one. This leads to three suboptimal outcomes. First, there can be an increase in uncontrolled infections, potentially followed by a recognized rise in the risk of immune system malignancies, and lastly, the cells can precipitate a condition of uncontrolled or chronic inflammation. The inflammatory process is associated with almost all chronic diseases of aging, including cardiovascular disease, arthritis, and neurologic decline. Therefore, this is a situation that must be addressed, avoided and/or reversed.

To continue the analogy, at the heart of any factory are the actual workers. These are the people that give the company its personality, provide the management and perform all of the hard labor. In our system, the real workers of the body are the actual, individual cells.

Real employees are usually brought in at the bottom, trained for their respective jobs, and cross-trained in some instances. Their work must be reviewed on occasion, and ultimately they are retired when the time seems appropriate.

Cells are, not surprisingly, the same. All cells originate from a mother cell, called a stem cell, that retains the ability to morph into just about any type of cell the body needs. To accommodate this, there are stem cells in almost every type of tissue, and they can provide replacement cells when necessary.

Stem cells, of course, live a long time. At the same time, some of the cells that they produce live comparatively very short lives. Skin cells and blood cells are prime examples of this, as they turn over constantly throughout your life. For example, you replace your red cell volume almost every three to four months. These live hard and die fast cells can only exist when the stem cells remain healthy and productive.

On the opposite end of the spectrum, some cells live an extremely long time and don't replicate or get replaced. Nerve cells in the brain, for example, are in this category. Most of your brain cells are with you from birth until death. They are tasked with not only thinking, but also controlling the rest of the body. Sensations, motor control, emotions- it's a lot of work! There are no fresh cellular recruits coming to the rescue, and cells can only tolerate so much stress. Therefore, when these cells get old, worn out and complacent, they have two choices. They can either commit cell suicide (apoptosis) or become senescent (retire).

Cellular senescence is like a working retirement program. The cell still functions, just not extremely well. They can make proteins and memories as they always have, for example, but frequently the proteins are corrupted and the memories are a little blurry. It is not uncommon for these cells to actually become toxic to the rest of the organism and thus become more of a liability. Because of this, there are surveillance cells that can get rid of such cells, but as we age, sometimes it seems better to have a poorly functioning cell than no cell at all.

The last category, but certainly no less important, is waste management.

Just ask the mafia!

Every factory has byproducts that must be tended to. Garbage must get recycled or ejected, or it ends up accumulating where it shouldn't. The body has such systems that under normal conditions are quite organized. Excess fluids are cleared out by the renal or kidney system, while solid waste is managed by the gastrointestinal tract. On a cellular level, however, most byproducts are recycled. Those that are not are then transported by the vascular system to the liver or kidney for detoxification, and then excretion.

But there is also waste that goes unrecognized and under treated. Excess glucose is one such problem. Glucose that floats around in the vascular system likes to stick to other molecules.

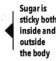

Sugar is sticky both inside and outside the body

This sticky, molecular glob, known as an AGE or Advanced Glycation End product, ends up destroying collagen and initiating innumerable, detrimental pathways. AGEs, for example, are a big contributor to skin drooping and heart failure.

The accumulation of trash actually occurs in every cell. If a cell is short-lived, the garbage gets taken out with the dead cell. Unfortunately for the long-lived cells, the garbage just accumulates. Therefore, over time, years and years in fact, there is a build up of garbage that the cell does not know what to do with. This build up, called lipofuscin, eventually clogs up the cell, leading to its demise.

Thus, the body works as a very complex factory, chugging along over the years doing what we expect it to do. But as is true in an actual factory, machines break, miscommunications occur, mistakes get missed, security gets out of control, employees become corrupt and disruptive, and the garbage builds up in the corners.

The following chapters are going to examine these phenomena in more detail and it's going to seem a little depressing. But only after understanding why things decline can we begin to reverse the process.

CHAPTER 3

BIOLOGY 101

To initiate the quest of understanding the theories of aging and the subsequent therapeutic interventions, it will unfortunately be necessary to review a bit of biology. Most people will be somewhat familiar with the generic cartoon of the cell and a few of its components from the 5th grade. Since then however, the understanding of the cell and its organelles has blossomed such that the complexity is almost overwhelming. However, I'm going to keep this as basic as possible.

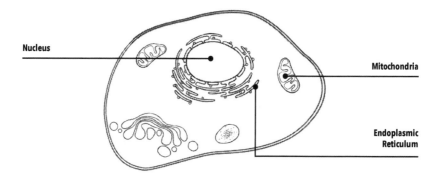

Nucleus

Mitochondria

Endoplasmic
Reticulum

The cell, regardless of where it is in the body and what it does, consists of a few very important structures.

The cell surface or outside barrier is a lipid bilayer (two layers) made up of hydrophobic and hydrophilic elements. The hydrophilic, or water-loving, sides face into the cell and out into the rest of the world. The middle of the sandwich consists of the hydrophobic, or water-fearing part. Embedded within this two layer, fatty membrane are hundreds if not thousands of proteins. These proteins can communicate information from the inside to the outside of the cell and back. They serve as carriers to transport goods across the membrane, and they participate in cell defense among other things.

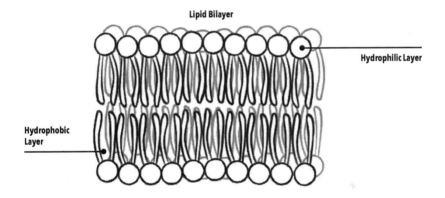

Inside the cell, the most recognizable organelle (little organ) is the nucleus. As the brain of the cell, the nucleus houses the DNA for the organism. This DNA serves as an almost complete instruction manual for the cell. As every cell carries a copy of the bodies total DNA, it seems intrinsically apparent that this is an amazing amount of information in a very small space. There-fore, it follows that like living in a very small apartment, the storage strategy is pertinent to survival.

In the case of DNA, Watson and Crick in 1953 described the classic double helix of repeating base pairs that resembles a spiraling ladder (There is a lot more detail in the Genetic Components chapter, so don't sweat it if your DNA recall is a bit rusty). This base strand, for the purposes of space and organization, is then wound around a cluster of 8 proteins (stacked 4 x 2) called histones.

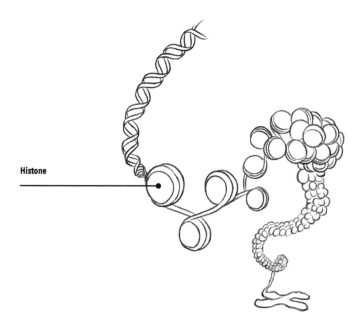

Histone

When the cell requires the production of a particular protein, a signal called a transcription factor is sent to the nucleus in search of the directions. Once located, the appropriate gene is unraveled so that the directions are accessible. This physical exposure allows for direct access to the correct DNA region by protein production mechanisms so that they can do their thing; but alas, my apologies…too much DNA information too soon.

The second most recognizable organelle is the mitochondria (aka the Mighty Chondria). This is the power station of the cell. The mitochondria has an outer protective membrane again made up of a lipid bilayer, and then a second, highly folded lipid bilayer where the energy is actually produced.

The organelle functions by creating an energy gradient across the inner membrane which converts energy in the form of food into a form that the cell can utilize, ATP. All along the inner and outer membranes, embedded proteins serve innumerable functions in terms of nutrient delivery, electron transport, oxygen management, and energy storage.

Again, more about this later. ▶

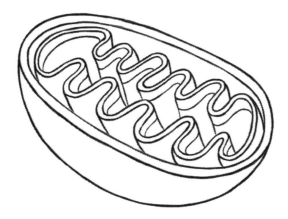

Mitochondria, once upon a time, billions of years ago, were their own independent cells. Then, at some point in time, they became incorporated into another cell in a very successful, symbiotic relationship. As a consequence or result of this, mitochondria carry their own DNA. This DNA, referred to as mDNA, is less in quantity that the nuclear DNA, but extremely important nonetheless. As well, nuclear DNA mixes under the conditions of sex and as a result, the child gets a mix of both parent's DNA. Mitochondrial DNA, in direct opposition, does not mix. The maternal mDNA gets carried down undiluted from offspring to offspring.

The third most important organelle is the actual protein factory. As all cells must produce proteins to survive, they do this in a tubular structure called the endoplasmic reticulum (ER). Much like a conveyor belt, the amino acids get put together into a complex protein as they proceed through the ER. The directions, of course, come from the nucleus. During the protein production process, there is a complex set of guiding proteins or chaperones that ensure the quality and functionality of each protein.

There are many other organelles in the cell, of course, but for now we are going to keep it simple.

CHAPTER 4:

INFORMATION SYSTEMS - GENETIC COMPONENTS

The first extremely relevant topic to aging is that of the genetic code. As discussed in the previous chapter, genes comprise the instruction manual for the body, in its entirety. Every instruction a body will ever need is pre-written. It knows when to start growing, when to stop growing, and exactly where said growing needs to occur. It dictates things that you take for granted, like having one head or a perfectly centered nose, as well as the minute details that make you, well, you!

The question posed decades ago when people first started thinking about aging, with respect to genetics was if there was a single gene, just one, that could control aging. Could we just flip a switch and turn it on or off? After years of extensive research, instead of that basic question being answered, the scope of the question just expanded. As is usually the case, discoveries don't actually clarify much of anything; they just uncover more complex questions.

But in the world of aging, time has proven fruitful. The first questions asked were if we could control aging. The clear answer has become, yes, we can - to some degree. The process isn't simple, but honestly, no one really ever expected it to be. There is no single gene that regulates aging, but there are a number of them that have been shown to be important.

As the years advanced, the study of aging and DNA stratified particular genes into categories that all contribute to this control process. Presently, there are six general classifications of genes associated with aging that we may be able to tinker with.

Don't worry, there are no pop quizzes!

1. **Life Span Regulators:** There are actually genes that act as life switches, of the on/off variety. These regulating genes are responsible for the sensing of external environmental conditions and cause the body to respond accordingly, which can either help or hurt the aging process. For example, caloric restriction (a 30% reduction in calories without starvation) is known to prolong lifespan for many life forms, including mammals. The body senses the environmental change, particular genes are activated, and the body slows down to conserve energy. The SIRTUIN gene family falls into this category and will be discussed extensively later. The good news is that we have the ability to activate this response without actually starving!

2. **Mediator Genes:** Think middle management - these are genes that receive the signals from the regulator (above) and serve to incite the production of specific proteins that actually alter cellular function (effectors). For example, if a gene needs to get turned on, the mediator produces either a kinase, protein deacetylase or transcription factor (Realizing these are new terms, I figured if I start throwing them out there, eventually, they will start to be recognized and make sense). These are specific proteins called enzymes that can mediate the speed of reactions. Like most mediators, the proteins that these genes produce don't do much on their own, but they serve as a middle or bridging step. Luckily, these factors can be manipulated to reach particular cellular goals.

3. **Effectors:** These are the action proteins; they do something tangible. For example, free radicals are a byproduct of

cellular metabolism that are quite damaging. In order to combat these radical byproducts, the cell produces its own antioxidants. Superoxide dismutase and catalase are examples of such effectors. DNA repair proteins also fall into this category.

4. **House Keeping Genes:** These genes act ubiquitously at every stage in the cell, because as in life, there will always be dirty laundry and dishes. These tend to support basic cellular functions. In this category, for example, there is mitochondrial upkeep, removal of the cellular waste or garbage, and loss of these functions usually limits lifespan and health span.

5. **Mitochondrial Function Genes:** Located in the mitochondria, these genes regulate energy metabolism. They control things like the electron transport chain and free radical production within the organelle. Loss of mitochondrial function and output is devastating to a cell, and it's encompassing organism.

6. **Cellular Senescence Genes:** These genes regulate the cell cycle. They are active in stem cell signaling at the beginning of a cell's life, and in the elimination of harmful cells. This extermination of cells gone bad is one way in which the body avoids cancer.

Taken together, the genetic control of the body and aging is controlled by thousands of genes. One of the best known longevity genes in humans at the moment is FOXO3A. This gene belongs to a family of transcription factors (in the mediator family) that effect insulin action and help to control stress resistance. In other words, the gene codes for a protein that attaches directly to a very specific piece on the DNA, and then transcribes or copies this information in order to make another protein (an effector) that then does the actual job.

Kinda like how your boss makes you do all his work!

There are several things to consider when pondering this gene. First, genes don't code directly for aging or not aging; they code for secondary actions that then contribute to the aging problem. Secondly, from this discovery, we have ascertained that insulin and thus glucose control and stress modulation are extremely important to lifespan and health span improvement. Therefore, other genes, products, events or proteins that have similar roles may effect lifespan as well.

Another gene demonstrated to promote longevity codes for chaperones. These smaller proteins accompany all significant proteins from production into action, making sure that they function as they are intended.

They also make sure no one spikes the punch bowl.

When such a protein malfunctions and has the potential to cause a cell harm, the chaperone makes sure it is disposed of properly. In this way, it serves as part of the quality control system. Much like the FOXO gene, the chaperone does not code directly for longevity. Instead, it is integral in the control mechanisms, which ultimately help in the quest for such longevity.

This discussion assumes that the DNA is in perfect working order; that every message relayed to the rest of the cell is pristine. Unfortunately, nothing is perfect. Over time and with every cell division, DNA is traumatized such that errors in the instruction manual slowly work their way into the cell.

Before a discussion of DNA failure, it would probably be helpful to take a small timeout and examine the actual structure of DNA. Without this, it probably won't make a lot of sense.

DNA, deoxyribonucleic acid, is an extremely long molecule resembling a spiraling ladder. Each rung of the ladder is composed of a deoxyribose sugar molecule with a phosphate making the side of the ladder, and a nitrogen base composing the actual step. On the other side of the ladder, you find the same thing, a deoxyribose sugar molecule and phosphate up the side but with a different nitrogen base as the stair. There are only four nitrogen bases: Adenine, Thymine, Guanine and Cytosine; and each one can only pair with one of the others. Therefore, at each step you will find either Adenine - Thymine or Guanine - Cytosine. It is the repetition of these combinations over a zillion times that comprises the real, actual DNA code. (Actually about 3 billion base pairs.)

This baseline 3D structure was discovered in 1953 by James Watson and Francis Crick in England as I mentioned earlier. By 1958, it was understood that when a cell needed to divide, the DNA doubled so that

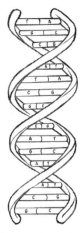

each cell would get a full copy. In order to do so, the ladder comes apart like a zipper, separating right down the middle. A specialized enzyme, DNA polymerase, then comes into the picture and helps recreate the missing side of the DNA. Thus, the DNA serves as its own template or mold. As there are only 4 nucleotides and one can only match with a set partner, the copying process simply lines up the pieces that fit. Thus, at the end of the process, there are 2 complete, and importantly, identical, copies of the DNA.

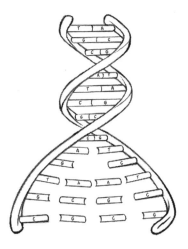

The next step in understanding DNA is realizing that the seemingly endless list of A, T, C and G's are actually an alphabet of sorts. A triplet of letters, called a CODON, codes for each of the 20 amino acids found in humans. For example, the pattern GGA denotes glycine. The strand of DNA can then be understood as code for a long list of amino acids, which when produced and strung in succession, create a specific protein.

This process is controlled by another group of molecules called RNA or Ribonucleic Acid. These come in various forms, i.e., messenger RNA, transfer RNA and ribosomal RNA and they serve as intermediates in the process. The RNA essentially takes the copied information out of the nucleus, into the cytoplasm, and into the endoplasmic reticulum where the protein can be manufactured.

In a more concise version, the DNA is the template, and the RNA acts as a mold to produce proteins.

Bet you're happy to see that 'concise' word!

Getting back to the structure of DNA, the double helix would be an extremely long molecule if left unwound. Therefore, it is packaged in a neat and orderly manner which keeps it organized. Ingeniously, the double helix of DNA is wrapped around a set of eight proteins called histones. These eight subunits, two each of H2A, H2B, H3 and H4, fit together in a neat square. The DNA is wrapped around each cluster twice, for a length of about 147 base pairs. A strand of DNA then turns out looking a lot like a string of Christmas lights with frequent, regularly spaced clusters.

With the Kaufmann Protocol, you'll have the energy to put these lights up for years to come!

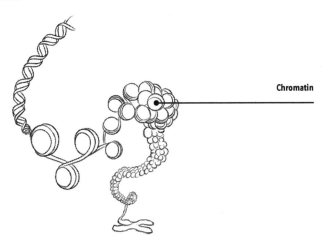

Chromatin

Next, this chain is bunched together in formations called chromatin. Tight chromatin is called heterochromatin, while less densely arranged chromatin is referred to as euchromatin. Because euchromatin is loosely bound, the DNA is more accessible to transcriptional factors and proteins, and is thus more readily available to be copied. Heterochromatin, being tightly packed, is therefore considered "transcriptionally silent."

The last item of importance to our DNA discussion is that of telomeres. Telomeres are simply the tail ends of DNA that code for essentially nothing. Once called "nonsense DNA," the telomeres were thought to be useless. Recent studies, however, have found a very high correlation between lifespan and length of telomeres, and thus a strong interest was sparked.

These repetitive sequences at the end of each chromosome may help prevent DNA deterioration or have something to do with cell replication-no one really knows for sure. But as we age, telomeres are known to get shorter and shorter as the cell divides and the DNA gets replicated. With each replication and each shortening of the DNA, it has been proposed that the ability of a cell to replicate is reduced. In fact, it has been estimated that we lose between 48-67 base pairs per year on average.

Like any important rope, you gotta tie a knot at the end! ▶

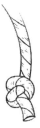

At the very end of the telomere, there is a knot of sorts that keeps things from unraveling. Made of 300 base pairs of DNA, the tail forms a T-loop which is then stabilized by specialized proteins called a sheltering complex.

• •

The 2009 Nobel prize in Physiology or Medicine was awarded to Elizabeth Blackburn, Carol Greider and Jack Szostak for identifying the importance of telomeres. They also identified an enzyme, telomerase, that actually can increase the length of telomeres in certain cells.

• •

Now that we are starting to understand at least the basics of DNA, the next question of course, is: What could possibly go wrong? Things going wrong is the basis of all types of diseases, appearing from early childhood and sometimes not manifesting until much later in life. Genetic diseases vary from sickle cell anemia to Parkinson's to even a propensity for developing cancer. And aging is no different, errors in DNA and it's processing contribute significantly to the decline in function and efficiency.

Therefore, I repeat the question. What could possibly go wrong?

Unfortunately, almost everything.

An individual's DNA is, of course, a combination of the maternal and paternal DNA as determined by the very first cell that was created when sperm met egg. The starting point of every individual is this one set of newly combined genes, which constitute the best the genes will ever be. It would be nice if this starting set were perfect, that is, devoid of any errors.

A perfect human is difficult to come by, and I've certainly never dated any!

Unfortunately, a vast number of people are born with incomplete genes, duplicated genes, or erroneous genes that prevent the organism from doing all it's required to do in an optimal fashion.

One error in one amino acid, for example, leads to achondroplasia, the most common form of dwarfism. Another single change in an amino acid leads to sickle cell anemia. Consider yourself fortunate if this was not your fate.

Beginning with this one set of instructions for the entire body, this instruction manual gets replicated over and over and over. It is truly inconceivable how many times the DNA gets replicated. And with any extremely good piece of machinery, usually the copy is perfect. Unfortunately, over time and with repeated copies, it is inevitable that mistakes occur. One simple exchange in a nucleic acid can lead to a single change in a codon, which can lead to an incorrect amino acid and thus to an incorrect protein.

A challenging environment can also cause degradation of the genes. DNA can get injured from radiation, chemical and even biological insults. Regardless of the cause, the production of an incorrect protein can lead to innumerable problems along the way.

Aware of this possibility, our factory has DNA inspection and repair systems. (There is a chapter on this a little later…it's an important subject).

These systems, made from proteins coded for in the DNA, probably catch a high percentage of errors. Regardless, over time, nothing is perfect (as we have come to realize) and errors will still occur.

What can one error do? It can do anything from corrupting proteins to precipitating cell death. It can incite malignancy. And worse than all else…it leads to aging.

Epigenetics

Once, it was thought that all of the genetic code was controlled by the base pair arrangement. More recently, however, it has been determined that there are a few layers of genetic control on top of this. These additional layers are referred to as Epigenetic, as they occur on TOP of the regular genes. As every cell in the body codes for every potential piece of DNA, it is the epigenetic detailing that controls exactly what each individual cell is going to specialize in. In other words, epigenetics is what makes a liver cell act like a liver cell, and not a brain cell.

Thus the phenotype (what traits get seen) gets differentiated from the genotype (what's in the genes).

For example, every brain cell and bone cell share the same genetic code, but the epigenetic component controls their different activities and phenotypes.

Epigenetics fall into a few categories:

1. **DNA methylation.** This refers to the addition of a methyl group (CH_3- one carbon and 3 hydrogens) to a DNA base pair. Methylation can only occur when a Cytosine is followed by a Guanine, referred to as CpGs. These additions are rather small, and tend to stick out the sides of the DNA ladder like lollipops. They serve to physically block the reading of that section of DNA. Thus, a cluster of methyl groups, as is usually the case, can look like Candy Land and functionally turn off a gene segment. In general, as an adult, about 4% of Cytosines are decorated with methyl groups.[1] As you might guess, this changes as we age.

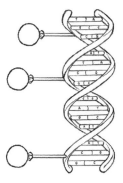

2. **Histone modification.** The histones, as mentioned earlier, are the protein complexes around which the DNA is wrapped. This mode of organization not only keeps the long chains nice and tidy, but also serves as a control method. Access to the DNA depends on whether or not it can unroll from the histone complex, and this in turn is dependent on the status of the histones. Over time, different types of "stuff " gets attached or removed from the histones, including the same methyl groups from above, or phosphates and/or acetyl groups. The addition of these molecules makes it harder for the DNA to unroll, thus limiting access to whatever information is encoded in that section. Different enzymes control the placement or removal of such blocking agents.

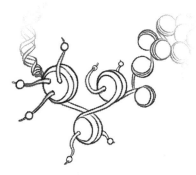

3. **RNA modification.** This is ridiculously complicated and not necessary for our discussion.

The question, of course, is why is any of this important?

• •

"Epigenetic modifications, potentiated by nutrition, have also been shown to delay the aging process, and certain changes within the epigenome have been adopted as potential biomarkers in many age-related diseases."[2]

• •

Like you didn't see that coming! ▶ This is crucial because the patterns of DNA modification change with age.

These alterations are referred to as epigenetic drift. We want our genes to control changes in our bodies when we are evolving from babies to toddlers to adolescents, but, when we are adults, we want the changes to cease. As the natural progression of DNA changes continue, we "drift" into becoming old people with increasing likelihood for cancer, diseases and just looking and feeling terrible. In general, with age, scientists have noted a global decrease in DNA methylation. In fact, total methylation is known to be inversely proportional to the maximum lifespan potential.

But more importantly than the total methylation, the pattern of methylation changes. Young DNA has distinct and dense areas of methylation, which become less distinct and more hazy with age. This epigenetic drift tends to vary substantially from person to person and the absolute changes are difficult to predict.

On the other hand, researchers have identified a set of very specific methylation changes that occur with age and tend to effect almost everyone equally. Credited to Steve Horvath and thus called the Horvath Clock,[3] 353 regions in the DNA that either get hypo (160 of them) or hyper (193) - methylated in a very time-dependent manner were identified. He determined that there was a very strong correlation between the DNA methylation pattern as found in blood samples, and how someone ages. Therefore, we now have an epigenetic or Horvath Clock that is extremely accurate.

• •

"Epigenetic drift is now understood to comprise age-related changes in the epigenome that include those that are acquired environmentally as well as stochastically."[4]

> *"In contrast, epigenetic clock sites show a relationship between age and DNA methylation that is consistent between individuals."[4]*

> *What can effect epigenetic changes? Chronic inflammation is the best characterized acquired modifier of methylation.[5] The actual mechanism behind this remains unknown, but the result is well documented. Unfortunately, the gist is that chronic inflammation, something that everyone gets with advancing age, precipitates drift which can then lead to cancer and aging. In fact, it is well known that cancer cells have a high degree of aberrant DNA methylation. Thus, reduce inflammation, reduce methylation and you in turn reduce aging.*

• •

Other known negative influences of epigenetic drift include chemical pollutants, stress, smoking, alcohol consumption, and UV light exposure. Generally, these are all the things that we knew were bad for us, but we were never really sure why.

It is thought that the drift in methylation patterns has a greater effect on cells that replicate more quickly. This is true for the lining of your digestive tract, for example, where the cells can replace themselves every 1 to 5 days. In this category, colon cells are known to have tremendous drift, and is hypothesized to contribute to the high rate of colon cancer.

Clearly, there are innumerable negative stressors on our DNA, but luckily there are also things that effect us in a positive way. For example, there are specific molecules in certain foods, that are known to be beneficial epigenetic modifiers.

Foods, you say? That's ridiculous. How can food effect your DNA?

Well, here is a really cool example: Honey bees within a hive are all genetically identical. The base pairs of worker bees and the queen are exactly the same, just like identical twins. The difference turns out to be their diet. All bee larvae are fed "royal jelly," a substance made in the mouths of nurse bees. But worker bees are cut off at some point, and fed pollen and nectar instead. The predetermined queen continues on the diet of royal jelly and thus becomes royal.

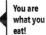 You are what you eat!

Therefore, the genes are the same, but the diet alters the epigenetics and thus which genes get utilized.

There are foods that are thought to do the same for us; not make us royal exactly, but positively effect our epigenetics. Taken together, they can be considered as an "Epigenetic diet." For example, curcumin is known to decrease DNA methylation as well as block histone hyperacetylation.[6]

"The term "Epigenetic diet" was coined to refer to the consumption of certain foods, such as soy, grapes, cruciferous vegetables and green tea, which have been shown to induce epigenetic mechanisms that protect against cancer and aging."[2]

Other substances in consumables thought to be useful in preventing epigenetic drift include:

- EGCG aka Epigallocatechin-3-gallate (green tea): *DNMT inhibitor

- Sulforaphane (cruciferous veges, esp broccoli, cabbage): DNMT inhibitor, **HDAC inhibitor

- Resveratrol (red wine, grapes): DNMT inhibitor, HDAC inhibitor (Activates SIRT1: a known HDAC inhibitor)

- Curcumin (turmeric): DNMT inhibitor

- Genestein (soy): DNMT and HDAC inhibitor

    *DNMT: DNA methyltransferase
    **HDAC: Histone deacetylase

• •

"Sulforaphane found in cruciferous vegetables, epigallocatechin-3-gallate (EGCG), found in green tea, genistein (soy) and resveratrol (grapes) are among the most characterized dietary compounds of the epigenetic diet."[2]

• •

These next foods are thought to be helpful, but details are sparse:

- Apigenin (parsley)

- Leukopenes (tomatoes)

- Butyrate (beans)

- Folate (green veggies)

- Boswellic acid (Boswellia)

- Selenium (Brazilian nuts)

- Quercetin (capers)

- B Vitamins

Some, but not all of these substances have enough evidence to be included in the protocol. The others certainly can't hurt you, they just don't help you as much as the others.

So, it turns out that the foods that your mother told you were good for you, really are. Fortunately now, there is proof.

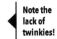
Note the
lack of
twinkies!

I did however say that this book was NOT about diet and exercise, so I can't actually tell you to consume these substances (Although it wouldn't be a bad idea). You can however, take them as adjuvants and supplements.

CHAPTER 5:

THE STORY OF MITOCHONDRIA

As we mentioned in the opening chapter, every factory is reliant on power. In general, energy gets delivered in a variety of forms, and then it is altered or processed locally so that it becomes more usable. As a real world example, coal, as a raw resource can be trucked in, and then burned to create usable electricity.

In the cellular model, raw materials in the form of glucose and fructose are delivered to the cell where it is converted into ATP, adenosine triphosphate, our equivalent of electricity. Every cellular function requiring energy is ATP dependent, making it the cellular energy currency. This transformation occurs in sub-cellular compartments called mitochondria which you may recall from the intro chapter. Second only to the nucleus, it is crucial to become somewhat familiar with this organelle as it is extremely intertwined with aging.

In case you slept through this chapter in remedial science class, I'm going to take a few minutes and review mitochondria; but don't worry, it's a good story.

Anyway...

Once upon a time, an extremely long time ago- roughly millions of years ago in fact, it is believed that a utilitarian yet beautiful relationship developed between two primitive bacterial cells.

Romantic already, right?

The bigger cell, utilizing inefficient and wasteful production methods was limited in its cellular functions by its energy requirements.

The smaller cell was more savvy and had developed an efficient energy system. In fact, it even had a power surplus; and so, like any good business takeover story, the larger cell took over or rather physically engulfed the smaller cell.

Not so romantic after all!

Now, the new even bigger cell had its own internal power generator.

As millions of years passed, this relationship became more interdependent (as most relationships do) and permanent (debatable). Today, all of our human cells are powered by mitochondria, the intracellular organelles which are the descendants of these smaller, energy laden cells. This proposition is known as the endosymbiosis theory.* First suggested in the 1970s, it is now generally well accepted by anyone that is remotely interested.[1]

As such, mitochondria can be conceived of as a cell within a cell. Structurally, they are usually oblong and capsule-like as is pictured in most diagrams, and thus will be here as well. They have one outer membrane and one inner membrane. The inner membrane is highly convoluted and thus has a relatively large surface area which is where most of the chemical reactions take place.

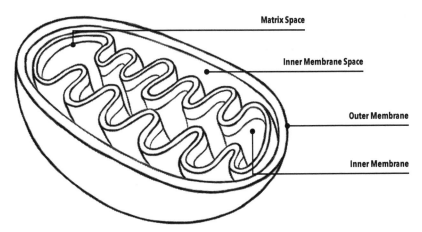

(endo=inside, symbiosis= work together)

In addition to understanding how an individual mitochondria functions, we need to understand that the organelles adjust and respond to the requirements of the cell in which it resides. These organelles can alter their shape, number, size and internal organization based on need. Depending on the energy requirement of a cell, there can be a few mitochondria per cell or thousands.

Mitochondria in cartilage cells constitute about 3 to 5% of the volume density, while in heart cells it can be as high as 37%.[2]

Tissues that have higher energy needs, like the liver, have between 1,000 to 2,000 mitochondria per cell. Oocytes, for example, start with 5,000 to 10,000 mitochondria per cell in the immature state, and rev up to 100,000 to 500,000 when they are maturing.[3]

• •

> *"The oocyte has, by far, the largest number of mitochondria, and mt DNA copies, of any cell, (approximately 2×10^5 copies), at least an order of magnitude more than somatic cells like muscle and neurons that have high energy requirements."*[4]

• •

These mitochondria increase their numbers by splitting in two, called fission. First, the organelle gets really big, copies its DNA and then divides. When a cell perceives a need for more energy, it responds accordingly. For example, when you initiate a new workout, usually a New Year's resolution, the newly challenged muscles respond by increasing their mitochondrial number and output. Conversely, when you quit the program in February, the mitochondria downsize.

• •

> *"Mitochondria are known to be highly dynamic organelles. They are able to divide and combine through the process of fission and fusion, allowing them to adjust their size, shape, and organization inside the cell."*[5]

> *"Mitochondrial dynamics are regulated during cell division, apoptosis, autophagy, mitochondrial biogenesis, and mt DNA integrity maintenance and are implicated in aging."*[5]

• •

Because mitochondria were originally stand alone cells, they carry remnants of this past.

Much like dating, there's always baggage

For example, while the cellular DNA is packaged as described in the previous chapter, mitochondrial DNA (also called the mitogenome, mDNA and mtDNA) is still double-stranded, but it is circular and thus has no ends and further, no telomeres. As well, it is completely separate from the nuclear DNA; that is, they do not mix at all. The mitogenome encodes only 37 genes and consists of a measly 16,569 base pairs. As well, mitochondrial DNA is passed down from mother to child pretty much unchanged over time.

As a result, mitochondrial DNA has been used to study evolutionary history…but that is a different subject altogether.

Secondary to having their own DNA, mitochondria are able to produce their own transcriptional and translational machinery for protein synthesis, or at least some of it. Mitochondria can't produce all of their own proteins however, as the average mitochondria has roughly 1,500 different proteins and these are encoded for and produced by the nuclear DNA. So, mitochondria have become semiautonomous and thus reliant on their home cell.

Now, back to morphology. The outer membrane of the mitochondria is reasonably smooth, consisting mostly of phospholipids and proteins.

Some of these proteins, porins (like pores or tiny doors), allow the movement of small molecules into and out of the membrane. Thus, ATP is free to glide in and out through the outer membrane unhindered. The space between the membranes is called the inner membrane space (not very clever), while the most inner space is referred to as the matrix.

The inner membrane of the mitochondria is convoluted as mentioned before, and is quite complex. In terms of length, the inner membrane is about 5 times that of the outer membrane.

The inner membrane creates a very strong barrier, separating harsh chemical environments and thus creating a chemical gradient. The only things that can pass freely are water, carbon dioxide, and oxygen.

Extremely complex protein systems called Electron Transport Chains are embedded within this membrane, and are responsible for the energy production. By virtue of pumping protons (H+ atoms) across the membrane, a chemical gradient is established. This is analogous to pumping water uphill in a slow, but steady manner. When the water eventually flows back down, the energy is recaptured. In the mitochondrial membrane, the protons, after being pumped across, are allowed to flow back into the matrix in a tightly controlled fashion that captures this energy and creates ATP.

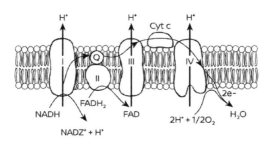

This gradient is driven by several spatially separated, protein formations that create a series of redox (short for reductive-oxidative) reactions. This is where an electron is transferred from a donor molecule to an acceptor molecule. Along the membrane, there are a series of these molecules, and as the electron gets passed along, it gets passed to progressively more electronegative molecules.

Think about a game of hot potato, but uphill

The final and most negatively charged receiver of the electron is oxygen. At the end of all this, the oxygen gets combined with hydrogens, and you guessed it, you get water. This game of electron hot potato is referred to as the electron transport chain.

• •

Reductive= gain of an electron, or decrease in oxidative state.
Oxidation= loss of an electron, increase in oxidative state.

• •

The electron transport chain is made up of many different substances that are imbedded in the membrane. Of note, coenzyme Q is one of these that receives electrons from NADH (a molecule you will soon come to love and adore) and passes them onto cytochrome C. In the popular literature, coenzyme Q has become a favored supplement for certain health issues. It isn't however, very important in the process of aging and thus it remains a footnote.

After establishing this powerful gradient, the protons are allowed to flow back through a protein embedded in the membrane called ATP synthase (synthase: "syn" means together. Thus synthase is an enzyme that puts molecules together.) This enzyme converts the gradient energy into biochemical energy in the form of chemical bonds by adding phosphates to adenosine. Usually there are already 2 phosphates attached (Adenosine diphosphate). This process adds a third, creating Adenosine triphosphate. This process, called oxidative phosphorylation, uses oxidative energy and acts to add a phosphate (phosphorylation).

Realizing this is a lot of information in a short space, I kindly ask for patience. We are getting closer to the part where things start to become important.

Inside of the matrix, the center of the mitochondria, several items must be present. The most important of which (for our purposes) are oxygen and NAD (Nicotinamide adenine dinucleotide). Succinate is also important, but it doesn't come into play for us, so I am going to leave it out.

Under usual conditions, the oxygen gets converted to regular water after accepting the electrons, which exits the mitochondria harmlessly.

Unfortunately, things never go completely as planned, and there is a small but reasonably steady 'leakage.' Instead of completing the cycle as they should, electrons remain attached to the oxygen molecules, making the oxygen highly reactive. This leads to the formation of several products, none of which are good. These include, but are not limited to, free radical superoxides, hydrogen peroxides, and hydroxy radicals- more about this a little later.

ALOT more!

The NADH also resides inside the matrix, produced by a system called the citric acid cycle. You don't really need to know this, but I have included it for the curious reader.

• •

The citric acid cycle, aka the Tricarboxylic acid (TCA) cycle or Krebs cycle, is a process used by almost all oxygen using or aerobic cells that utilize carbohydrates, fats and proteins as energy sources. These are converted into the energy precursor, Acetyl CoA. In a cycle requiring eight different enzymes, chemical energy in the form of guanosine triphosphate is produced, several amino acid precursors are created, and NAD+ is converted to NADH.

• •

The important thing to note is that the original proton that initiates the cascade of energy production comes from the conversion of NADH+ to NAD. This is key as the substance of NAD is going to become extremely important in our discussion about aging. Clearly, if there is a shortage of NAD/NADH+, the entire energy scheme falls apart.

With this basic understanding of mitochondria, we can look more closely at how time and aging can interfere with this extremely complex system. And then, even more importantly, we can begin the mitochondrial preservation battle.

Mitochondrial Superoxide Theory of Aging

As early as 1956, it was recognized that free radicals (an uncharged molecule or atom that has a single unpaired electron or any species capable of independent existence that contains one or more unpaired electrons) were created by escaped electrons during the process of energy production. The key add on however is that these are now known to cause significant harm to cells. Since then, this idea has evolved, taking into account new information about the inner workings of cells. We appreciate now that mitochondria are both the chief producers AND the chief target of free radical damage. It is also known that mitochondrial DNA is less protected and more exposed than nuclear DNA, and therefore accumulates more damage from these free radicals. At this juncture, the theory is referred to as the Mitochondrial Superoxide theory of aging.[6]

Why does this occur?

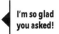

I'm so glad
you asked!

Let us return to the history lesson. When cells first evolved, oxygen was not very prevalent in the atmosphere. However, over the past 2.5 billion years as plants began converting carbon dioxide into oxygen, its concentration increased. Anyway, these once rare molecules became too numerous, and actually became detrimental. Cells did what they could to adjust, but the conversion wasn't perfect. As a result, the problem of free radicals developed.

As mentioned previously, the oxygen in mitochondria tend to attract loose electrons. This creates a pool of very reactive molecules that can cause significant damage to nearby proteins, structures, and DNA. These reactive molecules include: O_2^- (superoxide), $HO-$ (hydroxyl radical), O (oxygen singlet), H_2O_2 (hydrogen peroxide), and $ONOO-$ (peroxynitrite).[6]

It has been estimated that about 1% of all oxygen intake becomes a superoxide, and this percentage can increase up to ten times under conditions of physical exertion, which is why some studies have demonstrated that exercise can be detrimental to your health. One percent, under usual conditions, does not seem like that much, but over the course of decades, this can have a significant, negative effect.

The theory of aging proposes that these highly reactive molecules slowly destroy the cell from within. This can be envisioned as very small explosions occurring within the mitochondria. The internal and external mitochondrial membranes slowly get destroyed, leading to a deterioration in the proton gradient and thus a decline in energy production. The proteins also get destroyed, leading to additional malfunctions. In fact, all organic compounds can experience oxidative damage from this process.

In a downward spiraling cascade, the failing mitochondria then produces even more free radicals, and even more destruction ensues. Eventually, the mitochondria is retired from service and the cell produces a replacement. However, in its wake, the deteriorating mitochondria leaves the cell with extensive damage to contend with.

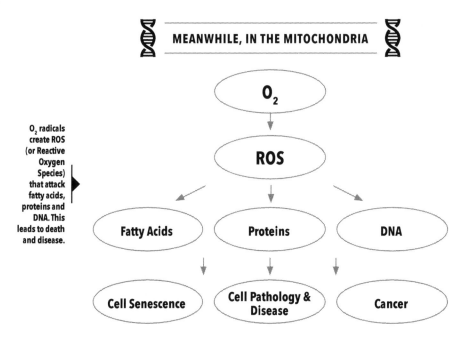

O$_2$ radicals create ROS (or Reactive Oxygen Species) that attack fatty acids, proteins and DNA. This leads to death and disease.

The importance of appropriately functioning mitochondria cannot be over emphasized. In fact, it is known that boosting the activity of mitochondria in small mammals can improve health span, reduce disease and even delay menopause in old, female rats. It has also been shown that if you can protect a cell against free radicals, you can improve the lifespan of an organism.

Realizing free radicals and reactive oxygen species sound like cellular doomsday, over the millions of years of their synergism the cell has developed mechanisms to cope with this challenge. To start, the cell produces its own antioxidant defenses which are capable of extinguishing the small explosions.

The first group of enzymes are the family of Superoxide Dismutases. These, in essence, dismutate or destroy superoxides. Discovered in 1968 at Duke University, they are metal-containing, antioxidant enzymes that break down the free radicals into oxygen and hydrogen peroxide.[6]

These come in several flavors, differentiated by the incorporated metal ion, and the localization within the cell.

1. **Copper/Zinc Superoxide Dismutase (SOD1):** The first identified, thus the "1," SOD1 is encoded on human chromosome #21, and the enzyme resides in the general cytoplasm of the cell. Often it is difficult to ascertain the importance of something until it's gone and in this case, the absence or reduction of this enzyme is linked to Alzheimers Disease, amyotrophic lateral sclerosis (ALS) and aging.[6]

2. **Manganese Superoxide Dismutase (MnSOD or SOD2):** This enzyme was discovered a little later, in 1973, and is localized on chromosome #6 in humans. The enzyme has a mitochondria localizing signal that sends the protein into the mitochondria after production. Unfortunate mice that are missing this gene live only 10-18 days and have serious issues with the heart, liver, skeletal muscle, and neurons. All of this implies that this protein is quite important.[6]

3. **SOD3 (Copper/ Zinc):** The active site of this enzyme also utilizes copper and zinc as does SOD1, but it localizes outside of the cell. It is located on chromosome #4 and reduced amounts of SOD3 are associated with Chronic Obstructive Pulmonary Disease (COPD).[6]

The SOD family reduces superoxides, but unfortunately it leaves hydrogen peroxide in its place. Whereas peroxide is less dangerous, it still isn't great to have lingering around in the cells. Therefore, glutathione peroxidase and catalase take over and further the conversion to water and O_2.[2]

4. **Glutathione Peroxidase:** There are 8 known versions in the family of human glutathione peroxidases, the most abundant being type 1 (as usual). Discovered in 1957, it is found in the cytoplasm of nearly all human cells. These enzymes contain the element selenium, which grants the molecule its antioxidant properties. Of note, GP 4 preferentially guards lipid membranes and thus protects against damage to the cell and organelle membranes.

5. **Peroxiredoxins:** There are 6 types of this enzyme in the human body, and they serve to break down hydrogen peroxide as well. Their most obvious role is in red blood cells. After hemoglobin,

which carries the oxygen, peroxiredoxin 2 ranks second in prevalence. In fact, mice lacking this enzyme develop severe hemolytic anemia (exploding red cells) and are predisposed to blood borne cancers.

I'm sure if it were discovered today, it would have a much fancier name! ▶

6. **Catalyse:** This enzyme is found in almost every type of organism exposed to oxygen, including bacteria, plants and animals. It was named in 1900, which explains its simple name. At the time, it was only known to catalyze a common reaction, thus it was named catalyse.

Anyway, this enzyme, as well, breaks down hydrogen peroxide to water and oxygen using iron as its metal. It is also super fast and efficient, and in fact it has one of the highest turnover rates of any enzyme. One catalase molecule can break down millions of H_2O_2 molecules every second.

• •

There is a theory that low levels of catalase contribute to having gray hair. High levels of cellular hydrogen peroxide are thought to bleach the hair from the inside, thus the inability to get rid of the hydrogen peroxide naturally bleaches the hair.[7]

• •

Reactive O_2 Species are treated by SOD, creating Hydrogen Peroxide. This is further broken down into H_2O and Oxygen. ▶

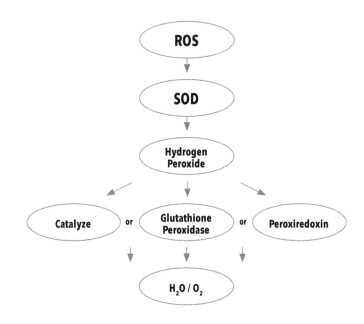

Therefore, every cell is in a constant state of flux; creating free radicals while protecting against them at the same time. Studies have shown that a small number of these molecules are necessary within the cell to aid in cellular communication. However, the vast majority cause disease and aging. So to recap...

Things that go wrong with aging so far:

1.   Sustained mitochondrial damage from free radicals or Reactive Oxygen Species (ROS) leading to reduced energy production.

2.   Decline in superoxide dismutase.

3.   Decline in glutathione peroxide.
        Studies have demonstrated a 50% decline in old rats.

Returning to the substances important in the mitochondrial matrix, Nicotinamide adenine dinucleotide has more recently been identified as extremely crucial for cellular preservation and thus aging. The substance is active throughout the cell, but as the first recognized role was in the mitochondria, we are going to discuss it in this section.

To start, Nicotinamide adenine dinucleotide (NAD) is exactly what it sounds like.

Two nucleotides, one with an adenine base and one nicotinamide, are conjoined by their phosphate groups. In the mitochondria, it is considered a coenzyme as it assists other enzymes in doing their jobs.

It was discovered in 1906, but no one had any idea of what it really was. The molecule, today, is known to be active all over the cell. It is part of the energy production system in the mitochondria; it serves as a messenger to the nucleus to assist in the control of mitochondrial activity, a cofactor to other proteins that repair DNA, and it is linked to sirtuins that help to control lifespan. In general, NAD plays several extremely important roles. Unfortunately, as we age, levels of NAD decline, while the need for it increases. The resulting shortage is thought to greatly contribute to complications with aging.

The molecule itself can be created by two methods. The de novo path involves eight different steps originating from the amino acid, tryptophan. This method is slow and requires a lot of cellular energy. An alternative, salvage pathway is also available whereby NAD can be recycled from nicotinic acid or nicotinamide. In most studies, it appears that the salvage pathway plays a more important role in NAD synthesis.

• •

In the mitochondria, most known activities of NAD are involved in energy production. In the TCA or Krebs cycle in the matrix, NAD is converted to NADH while Acetyl CoA gets broken down to carbon dioxide. NAD is also converted to NADH during the oxidation of fatty acids and amino acids within the mitochondria. The produced NADH then becomes part of the electron transport chain and is changed back to NAD.

• •

The point here is that a shortage of this molecule would be extremely detrimental to overall energy regulation, limiting several steps of energy production and thus mitochondrial survival.

In this mitochondrial-energy system, the NAD molecule is left intact (with the exception of the proton), and is thought of as a proton shuttle mechanism. However, our human factory has found ever more uses for this molecule. In several other cellular pathways, the NAD molecule gets used as a substrate, i.e., it gets broken down and its pieces used to create other things.

One of these uses is to assist in the repair of nuclear DNA. This is going to seem like a side trip, but it's important. I promise.

Poly-ADP-ribose polymerase, but more recognizable as PARP, is an enzyme that senses and repairs breaks in DNA. In the nucleus of the cell, PARPs role is to detect DNA damage, alert the troops, and then bind to the DNA and direct repairs. The repair machinery is complex, and depends on the actual type of damage that has occurred. The specifics will be talked about in the section on DNA repair mechanisms, but it is important to note that the initial step is recognition by the PARPs.

It turns out that PARPs need to create a chain of ADP-ribose units that get glued into the fractured DNA chain. These units are created by breaking down NAD, using the necessary pieces and discarding the nicotinamide.

• •

> *"The reaction catalyzed by PARP-1 uses NAD+ to form polymers of ADP-ribose units onto acceptor proteins, cleaving off NAM. Cellular poly (ADP-ribose) formation is dramatically stimulated upon DNA damage and, as a result, NAD levels plummet when DNA is damaged."*[8]

• •

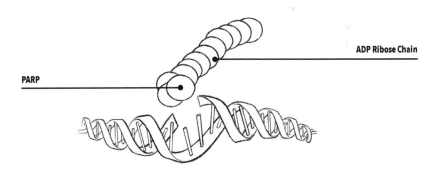

ADP Ribose Chain

PARP

Interestingly, PARP activity can be measured within cells, and its quantity correlates with the maximum lifespan of mammals; the higher the PARP, the longer the lifespan. Interestingly, even among humans, those that are long-lived have higher levels of PARP then those that are not. Families that have reduced amounts tend to be more prone to cancer. Therefore, it seems fairly evident that breakage of DNA is a reasonably common event, and the ability to repair the damage is critical.

It would also seem that the more PARP, the better things are overall. Unfortunately, this has been disproven lately and in fact PARP turns out to be a double-edged sword. High levels of PARP are good for your DNA, but it also increases the risk of metabolic diseases. It turns out that PARPs are pro-inflammatory. This makes many inflammatory based diseases worse, especially heart disease, diabetes, asthma, and fibrotic lung diseases among others.

Anyway, as we age, there is a known increase in DNA damage with the resultant increase in PARP activity. Using NAD to repair the DNA then leads to a steep decline in available NAD.

In yet another key role, NAD is crucial to the activation of sirtuins.[9]

What are sirtuins?

In reality, there is going to be a huge section on sirtuins in the near future, but for now, this is what you need to know.

Sirtuins are NAD dependent enzymes that sense environmental and nutritional stressors such as caloric restriction, DNA damage, or oxidative stresses. The activated sirtuins then trigger the transcription of specific proteins that enhance metabolic efficiency, increase anti-oxidant pathways (SOD for example) and facilitate DNA damage repair.

As such, many studies have shown that sirtuins promote longevity in mice, worms and most living things. High levels of sirtuins can also decrease the incidence of type II diabetes, cancer, cardiovascular disease and inflammatory diseases. In essence, sirtuins are good; again, much more later.

Because these sirtuins are NAD dependent, the absolute activity of sirtuins is determined by the presence of adequate NAD. As we age, we need sirtuins on an increasing basis, and thus we need more and more NAD. Unfortunately, a reduction in SIRT activity downregulates mitochondrial biogenesis, oxidative metabolism, a decline in anti-oxidant production and eventual cell death.

A third key NAD dependent system involves a system called the OXPHOS complex that runs the oxidative phosphorylation in the mitochondria. In addition to this, its production helps coordinate communication between the nucleus of the cell and the mitochondria.

The OXPHOS complex is made up of several pieces, some of which are manufactured in the nucleus, while some are made in the mitochondria. Under standard conditions and normal levels of NAD in the nucleus, the various pieces are made in the two locations, assembled and moved into the mitochondria. However, when the NAD levels in the nucleus are low, the production of the mitochondrial produced components slows down. When this occurs, energy production in the mitochondria declines and the cell suffers. There is a recognized age-related decline in the OXPHOS production and efficiency with age, and this is now believed to be secondary to the decline of NAD in the nucleus over time.[10]

Clearly, NAD becomes a hot commodity as we get older with many systems battling over the molecule. Unfortunately, all of the systems are important and thus the tug of war over which enzymes and processes gets enough NAD becomes crucial. Is there an answer? Of course; but you are going to have to wait for the chapter on NAD.

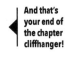

And that's your end of the chapter cliffhanger!

CHAPTER 6:

FACTORY PATHWAYS - YOUTH AND AGING

Now that we have addressed the informational and energy systems of our factory, we turn to the work flows or pathways. These aren't exactly assembly lines in the strictest fashion, more like metabolic dominoes. One thing happens, causing a second thing to happen and so forth.

Clearly my analogies aren't perfect! ▶

Regardless, let's get started.

So, over the last decade, a number of these metabolic pathways have been identified, and consequently dissected, that seem to exert control over organismal aging. We will examine several of these in this chapter, but first, the question is how scientists suspected they might be there in the first place. This is where that part of the story begins.

It has been recognized, at least in the scientific literature, for over a hundred years that caloric or diet restriction can influence both health span and lifespan. Skinny people (not starving, just thin) tend to be in better health, and live longer than their overweight counterparts. The realization that this was true for humans, as well as other organisms, initiated a recent frenzy in the anti-aging quest.

As a result, over the past decade, almost every organism that can live in a laboratory setting has been food deprived and their lives quantified. So far, caloric restriction (CR), as defined by a 20 to 50% caloric decrease from a standard diet, has been shown to prolong the mean and the maximum lifespan in dogs, rodents, worms, flies, fish and even yeast.

Higher up the evolutionary chain, the results are not so clear cut. Calorically restricted monkeys in one study lived longer, but in another they did not. Clearly, higher organisms are going to have more complex metabolisms with yet undefined confounding factors. Both studies did, however, show that caloric restriction increased the monkey's health span by reducing risk factors for diabetes, cardiovascular disease, brain atrophy and cancer. In fact, most animals on the diet demonstrated a delay in a wide array of age-related diseases including cardiovascular diseases and neurodegenerative declines.

Working up to people, the phenomena is harder to prove. There was an interesting study however, of Japanese folks in Okinawa in 1997. In comparison to the rest of Japan, apparently this subpopulation had an above average amount of daily physical exercise, a below average food intake, and lived longer as compared to other Japanese people. However, when some of these same families moved to Brazil, they adopted a less healthy lifestyle that effected both their exercise and food choices. Consequently, they gained weight and their life expectancy dropped 17%.[1]

So, following this train of logic, if we wanted to live longer we should just eat as little as possible.

Remember, this is not a book about diet and exercise!

Living on the edge of malnutrition, however, is not easy. Your social life would probably suffer as well would the rest of your body. Caloric restriction diets decrease fertility, libido, wound healing and the potential to fight off infections, while they increase the risk of osteoporosis. Perhaps starving is not the answer, but fear not, there is more to this puzzle.

As I stated before, not all studies support the association of CR to improved health span and lifespan, but most do in almost all species scrutinized.

● ●

"Caloric restriction with adequate nutrition is the only non-genetic, and the most consistent non-pharmacological intervention that extends lifespan in model organisms from yeast to mammals, and protects against the deterioration of biological functions, delaying or reducing the risk of many age-related diseases."[2]

"Caloric restriction is by far the most effective environmental manipulation that can extend maximum lifespan in many different species."[3]

The concept that "CR retards the aging process, delays the age-associated decline in physiological fitness and extends the life span of organisms of diverse phylogenetic groups, is one of the leading paradigms in gerontology."[4]

● ●

Questions then arise as to why this might happen, and then of course, how does this happen? Even more importantly, how can this information be utilized to help us?

To address the question of why, scientists have turned to the field of evolution. The going theory is that this response is an adaptation to preserve life in times of stress or famine.

The quest to understand how caloric restriction works initiated a new chapter in the study of human physiology. As a general overview, it was discovered that CR effects innumerable processes throughout the body. These range from affecting concentrations of various hormones, to the activity levels of different cell types. Most importantly however, especially for this conversation, scientists have uncovered several metabolic pathways that get either turned on or off under conditions of caloric stress that influence our time clock.

As time passes, even as I'm writing this book, new metabolic pathways and connections are being discovered that may or may not be critical to aging. For our purposes, however, we are going to focus on what I am going to call the 'big 3'. These pathways measure the environment in terms of stress level, nutrient availability, oxygen concentration, and then determine the best course of action for the organism as a whole.

AMP Kinase

The first of these pathways is controlled by an enzyme called AMP Kinase. Short for Adenosine Monophosphate-activated Protein Kinase, it's a central regulator of cellular and organismal metabolism that plays a critical role in maintaining energy homeostasis. It is otherwise known as the Metabolic Master Switch.

> *It has also been labeled a "fuel gauge" or the "guardian of the energy status."*

The enzyme is an intracellular sensor that acts exactly as it is named. It detects increased levels of AMP (and ADP), which means that the cell is in a state of low energy. Hence, this also means that the levels of ATP are low, as AMP gets converted to ATP when there is adequate energy. Once a low energy state is detected, the enzyme reacts by seeking out replacement energy.

Thus, AMP Kinase promotes catabolic mechanisms (processes to break things into smaller pieces) that generate ATP while simultaneously inhibiting anabolic systems (process that build different things) that require ATP.

This process is key to survival when an organism requires adaptive changes in growth, differentiation and process management under conditions of low energy. Whereas most cells have varying quantities of their own AMP Kinase, levels are highest in the liver, brain and skeletal muscle.

• •

> *"Efficient control of energy metabolic homeostasis, enhanced stress resistance, and qualified cellular housekeeping are the hallmarks of improved health span and extended lifespan. AMPK signaling is involved in the regulation of all these characteristics via an integrated signaling network."[5]*

• •

In a nut shell, the activation of AMP Kinase does the following:

In order to INCREASE the ATP production, the kinase:

1. Increases cellular uptake of glucose
2. Increases glycolysis, i.e. increases the breakdown of sugar to

produce more energy

3. Increases fatty acid oxidation, i.e. breaks down fats for more energy

4. Triggers the acute destruction of defective mitochondria while stimulating new mitochondria to be produced.

    This can be considered as a "cash for clunker" system whereby the cell recycles broken or used mitochondria to get more efficient, newer models. This is actually called autophagy, and will be discussed at length in a different section.

In order to DECREASE ATP utilization, the kinase:

1. Decreases fatty acid synthesis (essentially manufacturing less fat)

2. Decreases steroid synthesis

3. Decreases glycogen storage

4. Decreases protein production

5. Decreases cellular growth

In essence, the perceived shortage of energy puts the cell in a state whereby it can rebalance its own checkbook. It brings in energy from pre-owned fats and stored sugars, and ceases the creation and storage of more fats and sugars. The net effect here is the preferential loss of fat, and decreasing the storage of fat at the cost of growth and development.

• •

> *"It is known that AMPK stimulates energy production from glucose and fatty acids during stress and inhibits energy consumption for protein, cholesterol and glycogen synthesis."*[5]

• •

This pathway can actually be quite useful when exercising. When the skeletal muscles are stressed during training or a workout, AMP Kinase comes to the rescue. It increases mitochondrial biogenesis (creates more mitochondria), increases energy available to the muscle cells, and stimulates an increase in the blood supply to the muscle. Without AMP Kinase, the body would not be able to adjust to changes in workload.

There are also other housekeeping activities that have recently been linked to AMP Kinase, such as:

1. Influencing circadian clock regulation

2. Reducing oxidative stress

3. Reducing inflammatory markers

So how do these things actually happen?

AMP Kinase is a protein consisting of three basic subunits. One functions as the ON button (the catalytic unit); the other two initiate the processes. The ON button directly binds to AMP or ADP and alters the conformation of the rest of the molecule so that it can become phosphorylated, i.e., combined with a phosphate.

Once turned on, the molecule acts upon a number of substrates around the cell and around the body to effect change.

• •

Very little survives the process of aging unscathed, and the activity of AMP Kinase is no different. In fact, "emerging studies indicate that the responsiveness of AMPK signaling clearly declines with aging."[6]

• •

So, unfortunately as we age and the activity of AMP Kinase declines, this causes a growing number of problems around the body. For example:

1. Decrease in autophagy (intracellular recycling of proteins and organelles)
2. Increasing oxidative stress
3. Increasing inflammation
4. Increasing fat deposition (The annoying belly fat that

accumulates with age)
5.   Hyperglycemia (high blood glucose levels)

What usually triggers AMP Kinase?

1.   Low energy
2.   Ischemia (Lack of blood flow and resultant lack of oxygen and nutrients to an area)
3.   Anoxia (Lack of oxygen)
4.   Stimulation from fat-based hormones: leptin and adiponectin
5.   Exercise

Therefore, we have a situation where a necessary enzyme declines with age, bringing unwanted secondary effects that make the aging process even worse. In addition to this, the triggering list (with the exception of exercise) sounds rather unappealing.

The good news, however, and there had to be good news after all of this, is that we can pharmacologically improve the situation. The most famous of these compounds is metformin (glucophage). A well known and very common diabetic medication, it is also a mild inhibitor of the electron transport chain in the mitochondria and it precipitates a drop in the intracellular levels of ATP. The resulting increase in AMP triggers AMP Kinase, thus essentially faking an energy decline.

There is an entire chapter on metformin, so you will just have to wait to hear the other phenomenal things it can do.

In addition to metformin, there are several more natural compounds that trick the body into thinking it's starving. Referred to as caloric restriction mimetics, they also trigger the production of AMP Kinase. Clearly, it is easier to fool the body into doing the right thing than to actually starve one's self.

Caloric mimetics triggering AMP Kinase include:

1.   Resveratrol
2.   Pterostilbene
3.   EGCG
4.   Quercetin
5.   Curcumin

Not only will these be discussed in detail elsewhere, they also have innumerable other fabulous traits that you are going to come to learn and appreciate!

The Sirtuins

The sirtuins are another beloved family of genes and proteins that play a huge role in anti-aging, and thus constitutes the second pathway that we are going to consider. Otherwise known as the Silent Information Regulator gene, this family regulates the bodies metabolic and growth pathways. Discovered in 2000, it was noted that if yeast had an extra copy of the gene, SIRT1, they lived 30% longer than average. If they lost a copy (they would normally have 2), their lifespans would be shorter.

• •

As a side note (because it can get confusing), the genes are named in capitals like SIRT while the proteins that they code for are not, Sirt1.

• •

Much like AMP Kinase, the sirtuin family (genes and associated proteins) senses the environment in terms of energy availability, timing of daylight, environmental stressors and alters the metabolism to promote survival. Realizing this sounds familiar, sirtuin activity can directly and indirectly activate AMP Kinase activity, so many of the downstream effects are the same.

• •

"The close relationship between AMPK and SIRT1 is evidence that energy balance effectually controls cellular responses via an integrated signaling network."[5]

• •

Mammals (including people) carry the genes for seven members of the sirtuin family, cleverly named SIRT 1-7. The proteins Sirt 1, 6, and 7 tend to be localized in the nucleus, while Sirt 3, 4 and 5 are in the mitochondria and Sirt2 is in the cytoplasm.

SIRT1, discovered first and thus getting the #1 designation, is also the most researched of the bunch. The gene is located on the long arm of chromosome #10 (10q21.3) and the proteins it produces are localized in the nucleus, and thus govern the DNA. Like all of the SIRTs, it regulates the transcription of particular proteins, silences unnecessary genome sequences, and has myriad effects on epigenetic regulation. More specifically, it plays a role in the control of circadian rhythms, mitochondrial DNA transcription, the inflammatory pathways, and controls muscle wasting.

To make this easier, the following is a list of the genes (along with their personal information and effects):

SIRT1: Located in the nucleus

Circadian rhythm regulation (which is more important than you think)

Mitochondrial DNA transcription

Oxidative stress

Inflammatory pathways (NF-$\kappa\beta$)

Sarcopenia (muscle wasting)

Mitigation of metabolic dysfunction

SIRT2: Located in the cytoplasm and nucleus

Mitosis entry (cellular reorganization during cell replication and division)

Regulates fat tissue

Known to effect histones @H4K16 (thus an epigenetic modifier)

SIRT3: Located in mitochondria

Orchestrates mitochondrial function

Increases production of superoxide dismutase

Apoptosis (getting rid of useless dead cells)

Effects brown fat expression

Known to effect histones @H3K9

SIRT4: Located in the mitochondria

TCA or Krebs cycle (Controls cycle which is a preliminary step in energy production)

SIRT5: Located in the mitochondria

Uric Acid cycle (Don't worry about this)

SIRT6: Located in the nucleus

Controls inflammation through effects on NF-$\kappa\beta$

Telomeric preservation

Prevents diet-induced obesity

DNA repair

Extends lifespan

Known to effect histones @ H3K9, H3K56

SIRT7: Located in the nucleus

Controls nucleolar maintenance during cellular stress

As is readily apparent, this family of genes and consequent proteins are a well-connected and multifaceted family which you should get to know and respect. In the literature, the "sirtuins are now predominantly associated with government over longevity, disease prevention, and healthy metabolic function."[8]

The structure of the sirtuin proteins, while of course varying from one to the other, have 3 important conserved sites - the activation site, the NAD binding site, and the zinc binding site. There are two take-home messages here. First, there IS a NAD binding site, which means that the entire sirtuin family is useless without NAD. Thus, it is a necessary co-factor for the working function of the sirtuins.

As we discussed in the mitochondrial section, NAD was a rate-limiting molecule that declined with age, seriously effecting cellular energy production. The same deficit in NAD can devastate all of the vital standard cellular functions controlled by the sirtuins and especially their anti-aging properties.

The second take-home message is the zinc binding site. If you recall, the superoxide dismutase or SOD enzymes 1 and 3 also are zinc dependent. Therefore, it turns out that many micronutrients, like zinc, become especially important in order to maintain the innate anti-aging systems. Thus, micronutrient deficiencies can be catastrophic.

One of the most interesting, yet I believe under appreciated, mechanism is that of our circadian cycle. We take it for granted that we snooze incredibly well when we are young, and then struggle to sleep as we get older. It is yet another one of those things people consider inevitable. But, as it turns out, the circadian cycle is controlled by a combination of SIRT1 and NAD. Interestingly, both of these control and are controlled by aging; both decrease over time and luckily, both deficiencies are easily remedied.

The circadian mechanism itself is controlled by the production of four different protein complexes, two of which are active during the day, the other two at night.

The first daytime complex is the CLOCK, aka the Circadian Locomotor Output Cycles Kaput. Located mainly in the suprachiasmatic nucleus of the hypothalamus (a small area in the brain), this family of proteins is actually a complicated network of several proteins.

The second, daytime functioning protein family is called BMAL1 or Brain and muscle-ARNT-like 1.

Regardless, the two complexes work together and drive most of the oscillations in protein production in the body. Overall, they control up to 10% of the total transcribed genes.

The night time protein families are PERs (Period 1) and CRYs (Cryptochrome 1 and 2). These two work in conjunction to repress the activity of the first two. In essence, the circadian cycle is a constant battle with two against two. Interestingly, this process of inhibition by PERs and CRYs appears to be regulated by NAD.

In another bit of odd fate, the production of NAD is controlled by the circadian cycle, while the availability of NAD drives the circadian cycle. Seems a little inbreed, as well as a set up for failure. Regardless, having enough NAD is crucial.

SIRT1 and 6 control the activity of all four of the protein groups mentioned above. The take-home message here is that the loss of circadian rhythms with age is controlled by a combination of the decline in the sirtuin family in conjunction with the declining concentrations of available NAD.

• •

"Loss of SIRT1 in the brain not only regulates the circadian clock but also accelerates the aging process, which is most likely mediated by NAD."[9]

• •

The loss of sleep, a misery unto itself, is not the only problem secondary to the disruption in the circadian cycle. Metabolism and insulin production are tied to circadian rhythms, which makes diabetes even worse with age. Disruption in the cycle is also known to contribute to cancer. Women that work nights and have disrupted sleep are more likely to get breast cancer, and unfortunately for us, the rate of aging is also accelerated with the breakdown of sleep patterns.

• •

"Disruption of proper circadian timekeeping manifest in detrimental system effects and a number of clues from the clinic and laboratory suggest that these disturbances result in metabolic disruptions, cancer and age related phenotypes."[9]

• •

Another extremely important aspect of cellular control is the ability to effect cell division. In order to create a new cell, the mother cell must first replicate everything within itself, including its DNA and important organelles. These line up at the cells equator and then split evenly (hopefully) into two pieces. This cell division process is called mitosis, and occurs a zillion times daily in your body. Without activation of the sirtuins, however, the daily turnover of cells would be hampered; and without new cells, you aren't going to live very long.

Many of the sirtuins have also been identified as epigenetic regulators. As a reminder, epigenetic regulation is a system that controls what DNA sequences are physically available. This regulation can occur through DNA and/or histone modification.

Sirt2 has, for example, been identified as a histone modifier; more specifically a histone deacetylase. This is when an acetyl group is removed from a particular histone. Sirt2 effects H4 K16, meaning it modifies the acetyl group from histone #4 at the 16th lysine residue. Sirt6, meanwhile, acts at H3K9. By removing acetyl groups and changing the configuration of the DNA, the sirtuins serve as on/off switches.

• •

> *Most of the proteins produced by the SIRT genes are deacetylases, i.e., they remove an acetylate group from a lysine amino acid within a protein. (Thus they are mediator genes) Exceptions are SIRT4, which has only ADP-ribosyltransferase activity and SIRT5 which had demalonylase and desuccinylase activity.*[10]

• •

Whereas it certainly isn't necessary to know exactly what histone is effected in these processes, I think this type of information elevates the concept from the theoretical realm into a more concrete, metabolic intervention. As well, the proximity of the histone gives researchers an idea of what genes are being effected to further the course of study. But I digress; that is not our issue.

Regardless, this control is known to affect the key elements necessary for mitosis, which takes us back to the idea of cell division. SIRT2 contributes to the manipulation of tubulin proteins, which are tiny threads or tubes that push and pull stuff around the cell in order to get the cell ready for division. Think of all the little organelles like puppets having little strings attached. Thus without SIRT2, cell replication would be compromised, and, since NOT aging relies on the continual process of cell replication and renewal, this is a key mechanism.

My particular favorite thing about the sirtuin family however, is that several of them are able to preserve telomeric length. If you remember from the DNA chapter, telomeres are repeating sequences at the ends of the nuclear DNA that serve as protector caps. There is, in fact as we mentioned before, a strong correlation between length of life and length of telomeres. Therefore, anything that promotes telomere length has to be good. SIRT6, acting though histone deacetylation mechanisms as well, seems to be central to this phenomena, but admittedly, details are scarce.

Continuing on why sirtuins are good for your DNA, the last thing to note is that SIRT1 and 6 are important in the control of DNA repair. We are now very aware that DNA gets damaged overtime, so the repair mechanisms are crucial for survival. Also, remember that NAD is a necessary cofactor for DNA repair as it gets taken apart and physically placed into the holes as a patch. So NAD not only works in conjunction to drive DNA repair through the sirtuins, it is also used as a substrate to do the repairs themselves. Again, NAD is key to longevity.

This NAD seems to be pretty important!

SIRT1 also is known to trigger AMP Kinase. You already are experts on AMP Kinase, however, so I'll keep going.

Sirtuins additionally help to regulate the immune system, and as we well know (or will soon enough), chronic inflammation stemming from an out of control immune system is a huge problem in aging.

SIRT1 and 6 inhibit the Nuclear Factor (NF-κβ) system, which sits at the top of the inflammatory cascade. Thus, activation of this family decreases almost all of the inflammatory factors.

We haven't said anything yet about SIRT3, so let's have a look. Researchers at UC Berkley and Harvard have studied SIRT3 extensively in the mitochondria of hematopoietic stem cells. It turns out that the expression of Sirt3 proteins decline 70% from young to old mice cells. As well, the functionality of the proteins diminish by about 30%. This isn't surprising; it seems that all useful things tend to decay with time.[11]

They found that if you increase the expression of Sirt3 proteins in young mice, nothing happens. However, if you precipitate an increase in the Sirt3 proteins in old mice, many things happen- really good things! The production of superoxide dismutase increases, as well as its actual activity; this in turn reduces the mitochondrial oxidative stress. In the words of the researchers: "the more surprising finding of our study is that up regulation of SIRT3 rescues functional defects of aged HSC's (stem cells) and that oxidative stress-induced physiological stem cell aging and tissue degeneration are reversible." Thus, SIRT3 is particularly key to mitochondrial homeostasis as we age.[11]

One last interesting tidbit: SIRT1 controls the accumulation of white adipose (fat) tissue that accumulates with age. The less sirtuin proteins, the more the fat accumulates. Up regulation of Sirt1 in lab mice reduced fat storage, even when fed a high fat diet. This, in part, explains the abdominal tire syndrome that is so common in the human middle-agers. Of note, abdominal fat emits more inflammatory factors than regular fat. Luckily these can be blocked by the sirtuins as well.

Do sirtuins really play an actual role in life improvement? It certainly seems like they should! In lab mice that had over expression or extra Sirt1 and Sirt6, their lives were extended. As well, and maybe more importantly, they seemed to have overall better health. The mice demonstrated more physical activity, had improved muscle mitochondrial function, and slept better.

On the other side of the coin, mice that had less expressed sirtuins looked terrible and lived shorter lives. They had significant skin thinning, hair loss and reduced cellular regeneration.

So, after all of the research, I think it has become pretty well accepted that the sirtuin family is essential in the aging process. Unfortunately, as we all know, all of the sirtuin proteins decline with age, and thus, all of the age protecting mechanisms disappear with them.

Of course this all wouldn't be worth mentioning if there wasn't something we could do to boost our own SIRT activity.

Can anything increase sirtuins? Of course. Exercise is a key sirtuin enhancer, but I promised, this is not a book about exercise.

Caloric restriction also helps- feel free to starve yourself.

The best news however, is that there are readily available substances that are known to activate the sirtuin family. Of these, resveratrol is the most famous and it comes from red wine. But alas, there are many others as well! Stay tuned.

mTOR

Our third pathway of note is the mTOR system, and it is quite different from the first two. In fact, it actually seems to be in direct opposition. The mTOR pathway is essential for growth and development when you are young. However, as we get older, we just don't need it very much anymore. Unfortunately, the body just forgets to turn it off.

But I'm getting ahead of myself. Let's start from the beginning.

The story of the mTOR pathway begins, oddly enough, on Easter Island, thousands of miles out in the Pacific Ocean in the 1970s. In a soil sample taken in close proximity to one of the statues on Rapa Nui (the local name for the Polynesian Island), scientists identified a new anti-fungal agent and named it after the island, i.e., rapamycin. Isolated from *Streptomycin hygroscopic*, rapamycin has since been studied intensively for its immunosuppressant activity. The drug was approved in 1999 for use in post-organ transplant immunosuppression and is still used today.[12]

Since then, this compound and several of its derivatives have been approved for a variety of medical uses including the prevention of stenosis after angioplasty (the ballooning open of arteries), as a treatment for some cancers, and to treat autoimmune diseases. As interesting as this is, of course, this is not the reason we are talking about rapamycin.

While researching this medication, it turns out, scientists discovered a whole body signaling system that controlled cell metabolism, growth, cellular proliferation and survival. As you have determined by now, the naming system in science is terrible and uninspired, thus the name for this pathway became the "Mammalian or Mechanistic Target of Rapamycin."

• •

mTOR is a serine/threonine protein kinase, thus it's an enzyme in the mediator family.[13]

• •

This signaling pathway, much like AMP Kinase and the sirtuins, is influential throughout the body, effecting both intra and extracellular signals. It, as well, senses the environment, specifically amino acid availability, growth factors, insulin, energy status, oxygen levels and cellular stresses. In response, mTOR promotes anabolic processes; it builds things.

MTOR is essential to the biosynthesis of proteins, lipids, and organelles. This pathway is key to the growth and development of all cells and tissues, especially during the youthful periods of life. As a child and into young adulthood, growth is extremely important; in fact, I like to consider this system the pathway of youth.

Sounds better
than mTOR
anyways!

At this time, the metabolism of cells is high, cells grow and multiply, and new bloods vessels are created to provide nutrients to the new areas. This is called angiogenesis – think of new roads being built to supply new housing developments.

Unfortunately, as the body grows older, the need for unbridled growth is no longer important, and actually becomes detrimental. In fact, the pathway becomes obsolescent to a certain degree. It has been described as "an unintended and purposeless continuation of developmental programs which are not switched off upon their completion." Oddly enough, as the useful substances in the body decrease with age, the not-so-useful ones seem to increase, and so, mTOR activity, especially mTOR signaling in the hypothalamic neurons, increases in an age-dependent fashion.[14]

Let's examine a typical cell and see why this becomes a problem. In its youth, a cell sprints along doing it's thing; producing proteins and new cellular elements, dividing, communicating - its like a multi-tasking teenager.

As the inputs or activating stimulants start to decline, the cell starts to slow down. It still works, but it certainly doesn't need to divide any more. This is called "Cell Cycle arrest," meaning the cell stays in the same stage of life. It is equivalent to upper to middle life- the cell goes to work, does its job, doesn't complain, isn't partying all night and is generally content.

Unfortunately, mTOR does not want to leave these cells alone; the cells would love to revert to being more productive, but they cannot. The older cells simply do not have the capacity to respond they way they could before. As a result, these cells get pushed into what is called cell senescence. While these cells cannot divide, they begin to physically expand, and over produce whatever it is they were producing in the first place. The cells thus first become hyper-functional; homeostasis is altered, and age-related diseases begin to appear. Ultimately, they start producing inflammatory factors and begin inflicting damage to the organism.

Increased blood pressure, for example, is partially the result of the hyper-functioning of smooth muscle cells within the arteries. Platelets, responsible for the formation of clots when you are bleeding, become hypercoagulable and cause clots when they shouldn't. This can cause heart attacks and strokes.

Osteoporosis is the result of overzealous osteoclasts in the bone (osteoclasts destroy bone while osteoblasts rebuild bone…more on this later). Further examples include hyperglycemia, increased resistance to hormones, and higher circulating inflammatory factors.[14] As time passes, these processes eventually lead to cell death, organ and tissue death and then organismal decline.

Autophagy is another key concept we need to discuss (We will talk about this more in detail later, but for now here are the basics). The word means exactly what it seems to, "self-consuming or to eat oneself." This is an intracellular process where damaged organelles and unwanted molecules get broken down and recycled to make new ones. Removing damaged parts and pieces within a cell is crucial. Otherwise, cells end up looking like garbage depots or junk drawers, and cannot function as they need to. The other key purpose of autophagy is increasing the availability of nutrients when primary resources are scarce, i.e., it makes sense to recycle a broken mitochondria to make a new one. On the other hand, if nutrients are plentiful, the old mitochondria is left to rot and a new one is produced to take over its job.

MTOR prevails in times of high nutrient availability. Thus, it has no use for recycling. Activation of mTOR therefore blocks the process of autophagy. Conversely, blocking mTOR facilitates autophagy.

Research has demonstrated that blocking the mTOR pathway is good for longevity. This has been shown to be valid in yeast, nematodes, fruit flies, and mice. Blocking mTOR also seems to have some of the features of caloric restriction and in fact dietary restriction has been demonstrated to reduce mTOR. This makes sense if you think about it. If there are fewer calories to burn, the body should be conserving them and not actively growing. Along a similar vein, the activation of AMP Kinase, which occurs when nutrients are low, inhibits mTOR as well.

Blocking mTOR not only has theoretical advantages in longevity, it has also been shown to improve health span. In mice rapamycin studies, spontaneous tumors and cancers were significantly reduced. In addition, age-related declines such as changes in heart function, liver and adrenal function and endometrial changes occur much more slowly in mice treated with mTOR blockers.[15]

Rapamycin

As the keynote blocker of mTOR, rapamycin had been studied extensively and does some pretty incredible things. In innumerable studies to date in mice and rodents, rapamycin has conclusively elongated lifespan. The details of such include the following:

1. There is a delay in the loss of stem cell function. This is useful as tissues that require high cell turn over, like blood or skin cells, can make new cells for a longer period of time before pooping out.
2. Delay in cognitive decline
3. Delay in onset of retinopathy
4. Delayed heart failure
5. Delayed liver degeneration
6. Delayed endometrial hyperplasia
7. Less tendon stiffening
8. Less decline in physical activity
9. Cancer prevention (Being used at present for Renal Cell Carcinoma)[15,16,17]

All of these things are amazing and obviously what we all desire. Which, unfortunately, brings us to the saddest part of this journey; rapamycin comes with some terrible side effects.

For one, the drug is an immunosuppressant. That means that the risk of getting infections is extremely high. Mice and rats living in very clean laboratories don't usually have this as an issue, but as actual people, this would be a real problem.

Renal transplant patients on the medication report edema (swelling) (60%) and aphthous ulcers (55%).

Ninety percent of people lose their hair (alopecia), and most report other hair and nail problems.

Men lose testicular function and fertility.

In addition to these issues, there are a host of metabolic changes as well, such as hyperlipidemia, decreased insulin sensitive, glucose intolerance, new onset diabetes, and diarrhea.

Based on this list, it seems unlikely that normal people are going to sign up for this treatment. On a redeeming note, because I can't leave a chapter on a depressing bit of information, there is some good news. Metformin (glucophage), a drug we have mentioned briefly, acting through the activation of AMP Kinase can help to depress the levels of mTOR. It's not the perfect answer, but I'm sure we will find one eventually.

CHAPTER 7:

THE MAINTENANCE DEPARTMENT - QUALITY CONTROL

Following our factory model, we now turn our attention to when things break or malfunction. It's not the most upbeat topic, but it is an essential piece of the aging puzzle.

In any factory, as you are probably aware, infrastructure falls apart. Equipment fails, assembly lines get stuck, sinks get clogged, etc. You get the idea. The factory can deteriorate all by itself over the course of time, but it is also affected by the environment in which it sits. If your factory is in a flood zone, for example, you might be in trouble after a big rain. If you are in a desert, the dry air can desiccate parts that require moisture. The point here is that time is kind to nothing, and regular upkeep is mandatory.

Thus, every factory has a maintenance department. Scheduled, regular maintenance checks are standard, and repairs are a continuous, ongoing activity. In a new factory, less stuff breaks in general. The pipes are still clean, and the floors still shiny. Over time however, as the plumbing and the wiring gets old, things break more commonly.

Our cells are the same. When we are young, cell processes run efficiently.

There is day to day maintenance, but there isn't yet a backlog of things to repair. The exposure to insults is minimal. Skin is still flawless and tight, vision still precise, and energy is plentiful. Over time, however, the exposure to both internal and external forces grows and the damage accumulates. Cells have pretty ingenious methods to overcome a lot of this damage, but slowly and surely, the damage leads to the demise of function.

All sorts of things in the cell get damaged with age, but most importantly we are going to focus on DNA and proteins. We know for a fact that DNA damage accumulates with time, and surprisingly it is rather a lot faster than you might think. The good news is that every cell has extensive surveillance and repair systems. The bad news is, of course, that these systems get overwhelmed.

The same holds for proteins. Protein production in the cell is key to its very existence, and us, by extension. The cell is made of proteins, protected by proteins, repaired by proteins and oh by the way, they produce proteins for export. It follows that, like any good investor, the cell puts a lot of energy into controlling the quality of the proteins it produces. Therefore, every cell has a complex quality control system for proteins, and this system works... usually. It, like everything else, however, gets impaired with age.

But enough of the introduction. Let's plunge into the details.

To review a bit about DNA, you might want to flip back to the intro chapter on DNA.

Or at least glance at the pretty pictures?

DNA is a double helix, or a spiraling ladder, made up of base pairs. These chains are extremely long, and thus are packaged neatly by being wrapped around histones and then squished together.

Sort of

This DNA can get damaged in many ways. If the entire ladder breaks apart, it is known as a double-stranded break. On average, in every cell, there are about ten double-stranded breaks per day.[1]

If a single strand breaks, this is obviously a single-strand break. This occurs much more commonly, at a rate of about 5,000 breaks per cell per day.[2]

Innumerable other things can go wrong as well. This is especially true during cell replication when DNA gets copied in its entirety; errors are plentiful and can be classified as substitution errors, deletions, inter-strand crosslinks… you get the idea.

Overall, the adage that anything that can go wrong, will go wrong, holds true. Thus, inclusively, it is estimated that there are 10^4 to 10^5 DNA problems per cell per day.

Why does this happen?

DNA, in general, is fragile, and it comes under attack from many enemies. There are mutagens everywhere including ultraviolet light from the sun, chemicals, X-rays, and gamma irradiation as well as chemotherapeutic drugs. DNA damage can also occur from toxins the cell produces itself, namely the reactive oxygen and nitrogen species or free radicals that we discussed previously.

• •

"Endogenous sources for DNA damage include replication and combination errors (rate 10^{10}/bp), spontaneous hydrolysis, and reactive metabolites created as a byproduct of cellular metabolism like reactive oxygen species."[1]

"Double-stranded breaks have been studied extensively and are known to arise from ROS, gamma irradiation, mechanical stress, defective telomere processing, chemotherapeutic drugs and replication fork collapse."[1]

• •

So, knowing our DNA is constantly under attack, the maintenance department works around the clock. Once damage is sensed, the first response is to halt the cell cycle. If this damage is occurring while the cell is replicating, it certainly does not want to pass along the error to the next generation of cells. Therefore, all activity is blocked until the repairs are completed. Seems sensible.

Because scientists love identifying steps, they have divided this system into four main pieces: damage sensors, signal transducers, repair effectors, and cell arrest or death effectors. In normal lingo, this would be 1) identifying a problem, 2) sharing that information with the higher ups, 3) repairing it as well as possible and 4) dealing with the consequences.

• •

> *All of this together is called the DNA Damage Response system or the DDR. In all, it is made up of more than 50 different proteins recruited to the damaged DNA site.*[2]

• •

Recognition of the DNA damage is the first step. This is carried out by a protein family called PARPs which stands for Poly ADP-ribose polymerases. This sounds like quite a mouthful, but it describes exactly what it is. This enzyme glues together many (poly) ADP-riboses. We talked about this a bit in the mitochondrial section, if you recall, because PARPs are voracious consumers of NAD. The enzyme deconstructs the NAD molecule, pieces together the ADP-riboses, and discards the nicotinamide. In essence, it creates a chain that can be used as filler to repair the section of damaged DNA.

Humans are presently thought to have 17 types of PARPs that serve innumerable functions in the cell, some beneficial and some not (for our purposes at least). PARPs were first discovered, however, in the DNA damage repair system, so this is what we are going to address. PARP1, accounting for about 90% of PARP function, attaches itself to the damaged DNA chain and then dictates how best to repair the problem.

Because there are numerous types of DNA damage, there are several types of repair systems that specialize in the various anomalies. It is the job of PARP to activate the appropriate system.

1. **Base excision repair (BER):** This is the most basic repair system and deals with single lesions or small alterations of bases. It is usually a single strand problem, but it still consists of a large network of repair proteins.

2. **Nucleotide excision repair (NER):** This process excises bigger or bulky pieces of bad DNA. This is especially important in sun or UV damage, and I'll get to it in a second. Anyway, NER consists of 9 major proteins including enzymes like DNA

polymerase, DNA ligase, etc. Of note, studies have shown that deficiencies of these proteins are known to lead to premature skin aging.

As a side note, we now know that telomere length is, in part, maintained by the same NER pathway. Therefore, any damage to the NER pathway will also prevent the maintenance of telomeres, adding to the aging problem.

The following two repair systems deal specifically with the double-strand breakage, the most serious of the DNA injuries.

3. **Homogenous recombination:** Again, this repairs double-stranded breaks. Without going into details, it is a more laborious and energy requiring process, but overall it is extremely accurate.

4. **Non-homogenous recombination:** These also repair double-stranded breaks. This process is more like patching a flat instead of getting a new tire. It's a faster method, less energy intensive, but fraught with inaccuracy.

Despite the fact that most of you are hearing about this for the first time, scientists have been studying this stuff rather extensively for years. In fact, in 2015, three separate Nobel prizes were awarded for DNA repair system recognition.

So, what happens if these things don't work?

• •

"These lesions, if not correctly repaired, will interrupt genome replication and transcription and cause wide-scale chromosomal aberrations that trigger malignant transformation or cell death."[2]

"Dysregulation of DDR and repair is closely associated with human diseases such as cancers, cardiovascular disease, neurodegenerative disorders and aging."[2]

• •

The gist is that when the repair systems fail, the body does not do well. In fact, DNA errors are closely associated with the development of cancer.

When a cell's DNA goes rogue, sometimes there is no stopping it. Ironically, sometimes the DNA Damage Response proves to be a double-edged sword. For normal cells, it acts as a protective guardian of the genome. However, if a cell becomes cancerous, a highly developed DDR mechanism will allow that particular cell to develop resistance to chemotherapy and radiation.

• •

> *"Insufficient DNA repair mechanisms are also linked with cardiovascular disease and neurodegeneration. In specific, they play a role in such diseases as Alzheimers, Huntington's, and Parkinson's."*[2]

• •

Beyond cancer and other diseases, which of course we are trying to avoid, we are most concerned with how DNA damage causes aging.

How does DNA damage cause aging?

1. DNA damage causes cells to become senescent or die. If the DNA gets repaired, then all is well. If however, the repair does not work, the cell has to decide if the damage is serious or not. If deemed irreparable, the cell either undergoes apoptosis (death) or becomes senescent. A senescent cell, as will be discussed extensively in a different chapter, is not a good thing. It is a bitter, spiteful cell that exudes inflammatory factors and damages the entire organism. A dead cell, meanwhile, isn't any good either.

2. Senescence depletes the pool of stem cells. As stem cells are the busiest cells in terms of cell turnover and DNA replication, they are most likely to encounter DNA damage that is not repairable. Thus, over time, the pool of stem cells becomes diminished. With limited ability to replenish cells when needed, ultimately, the tissue in which they reside degenerates, and that particular organ fails.

3. Senescence causes chronic inflammation. I mentioned this in number one, but it's worth emphasizing. Chronic inflammation is a huge problem in the world of aging. Thus, anything contributing to inflammation is bad.

The other thing that helps us to understand the link of DNA damage to aging comes from a few rare and terrible conditions. For example, there are a few congenital diseases that consist of mutations in the genome maintenance genes. Referred to as DNA repair deficiency syndromes, these are characterized by developmental impairment, increased cancer susceptibility and of course, accelerated aging.[3]

The most studied causal link between the environment, DNA damage and the resulting tissue deterioration is in the skin. Therefore, let's take a small side trip.

The appearance of unwanted lines and discoloration, sagging skin, and excessive dryness all are signs of aging, and the vast majority of these problems stem from solar radiation. The skin, the largest organ of the body, is roughly 1.5 to 2 meters^2. So, not only are skin blemishes quite noticeable, the problem is extensive. Thus, the skin is an excellent model for examining how the environment can inflict damage upon us.[4]

Of the types of radiation that affect us the most, we need to consider UVB and UVA. At the moment, UVC is blocked by the ozone layer and doesn't reach the ground. This may be a problem for the next generation, but for now, we don't have to worry about it.

UVB (wavelengths of between 280-320 nm) represents about 5% of solar radiation that reaches us and it penetrates the entire epidermis and into the dermis.

What is interesting about UVB radiation is that it directly attacks the DNA. In fact, the DNA absorbs its photons readily and this causes very specific defects in the strand.

Cyclobutane pyrimidine dimers (CPD's) and pyrimidine pyrimidones are such complexes that form when the DNA is sort of 'melted together.' This forms bulky, distorted regions in the double helix that require repair by the NER system. The specifics of this aren't too important, except that scientists can directly measure the damage inflicted by UVB damage, and it is impressive.

In addition to the direct damage to DNA, UVB radiation also causes an increase in oxidative stress. There are inherent systems in the skin to combat these free radicals, but excessive exposure overwhelms and depletes the cutaneous defense system. This, over time, leads to extensive photoaging.

• •

> *"UVB radiation can induce both direct and indirect adverse biological effects including the induction of oxidative stress, DNA damage, premature aging of the skin."*[2]

• •

On top of photoaging, UVB radiation is also known to cause both melanoma and non-melanoma type skin cancers.

UVA radiation (wavelengths 320-400 nm) constitutes much more of the solar radiation that reaches us, about 90 to 95%. Known as the 'aging ray,' it penetrates through the epidermis and much farther into the dermis. The damage inflicted by this radiation is almost entirely though the production of singlet oxygen and free radicals. As we have learned from other chapters, these free radicals trigger extensive damage to proteins, lipids, as well as DNA. This particular DNA damage is different from that caused by UVB radiation, and can be measured by the production of 8-oxo-7,8-dihydro-2-deoxyguanosine (and similar type molecules), a damaged component of the DNA.

Protection against UVA radiation includes the endogenous antioxidant pathways, and when that fails, the lesions get repaired by the BER system.

• •

> *"In contrast to UVC or UVB, UVA is barely able to excite the DNA molecule directly and produces only a small number of pyrimidine dimers in the skin; therefore it is assumed that much of the mutagenic and carcinogenic action of UVA radiation is mediated through reactive oxygen species."*[2]

• •

As a side note, there is a great study demonstrating that UVA generated ROS are involved in the depletion of skin melanocyte stem cells. As a consequence of this loss, rather than the production of colored hair, gray hair is produced instead. Thus, protecting your DNA may also preserve your hair color.[2]

What to do about the damage from radiation? Sun block is of course key, but almost more important is maximizing the antioxidant capability of the skin.

The good news is that can readily be accomplished.

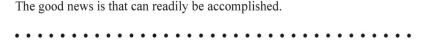

"Currently, prevention and treatment strategies for photo-aged skin mostly center on strengthening antioxidant defense for the cells."[2]

The various DNA repair processes that we've discussed rely, of course, on appropriately functioning proteins. Thus, in order to preserve DNA structure and function, we need to next address the protein quality control systems.

Protein repair

Before we understand why protein homeostasis is so important, let's take a minute and review exactly what proteins are. I'm sure most people use the term when referring to food, but for our purposes, it needs to be a little more specific.

Cellular proteome: the entire pool of proteins located inside cells and in their plasma membrane

Proteins, at their most basic level, are simply chains of amino acids. There are probably over 500 amino acids in the world, but there are only 20 in the human protein world. The order of the specific amino acids that make up a protein is determined by the genetic code. This information gets translated through codons, as we learned much earlier. This chain is built in the endoplasmic reticulum, which serves as a moving assembly line. As the chain is constructed, it is folded into a unique, three dimensional structure that is necessary for its biological function.

These proteins, once manufactured, remain very dynamic. They undergo frequent conformational changes with partial to complete unfolding and refolding to translocate across membranes, and assemble into functional units.

When we speak broadly about proteins, the other thing to remember is that proteins have many roles. In factory terms, the proteins constitute the assembly line itself, as well as the widgets made on that assembly line.

As we saw with DNA, when things are working smoothly, all is well. However the damage inflicted upon the protein system over time is unending. In fact, of all the molecules to be attacked or negatively effected by ROS, 70% are proteins. Of note, the most vulnerable are those that contain sulfur side groups. Therefore, in order to both avoid, but then to consequently repair damage to proteins, very intricate systems are in place.

The first such mechanism is the chaperone system. Chaperones, small proteins unto themselves, accompany the other larger proteins throughout their proteinaceous lives. The chaperones duty is to protect the protein as it morphs into different shapes and guard it from attack when it is vulnerable. For example, when a protein unfolds, it is like exposing a soft underbelly. The protein can't protect itself from any onslaught of molecular enemies. It is therefore the task of the chaperone to protect its protein and then help to refold it when necessary.

Unlike a human chaperone that gets to retire when their kid is of age, the molecular chaperone stays with its protein its entire life. It is, in essence, more like a bodyguard or personal assistant.

There are hundreds of these chaperones known in our bodies, and they are highly conserved throughout nature. Meaning, our chaperones look a lot like those found in common bacteria. For those curious geeks, these molecules are classified by molecular weight of which there are five groups. They are also described by the particular cellular compartment in which they reside. These details aren't really necessary, except to note that cells invest tremendous energy in protecting their proteins. Unfortunately, the quantity and quality of some, but not all, chaperones are known to decline with age.

When one of these chaperones fails in its duty and a protein goes rogue, special teams gets activated. Proteins can also be defective from their very inception, again mandating the activation of a special service.

The cell's first attempts are geared toward repairing the damaged protein. Depending on the degree of deterioration, this can be either successful or not. When this fails however, the bad protein must be eliminated. It is then taken to the proteolytic department and destroyed.

This deconstruction process is accomplished by the Ubiquitin/ Proteasome system or the UPS. Among several less extensive protein surveillance and destruction services, this is the major cellular system for selective removal of damaged proteins. In other words, it holds the monopoly on waste management services.

Conveniently, ubiquitin proteins are ubiquitous! ▶ This system works in two stages. First, bad proteins are identified and tagged. Labeling consists of the addition of a small protein called a ubiquitin. More ubiquitins get progressively added to the first, with the eventual formation of a poly-ubiquitin chain. Thus, the bad protein is labeled with an extensive tail. This complex is then taken away and destroyed.

What can brown do for you? ▶ As we have come to realize, all systems fail with age. The UPS system is no different.

• •

> The UPS "*undergoes age-dependent changes that contribute to the lower efficiency of this system in old organisms and the consequent alterations in proteostasis.*"[5]

• •

So, why is protein failure important? Why does this cause us to age? Two reasons, really.

Number one: the loss of function. If a cell can't manufacture the required proteins, it can't perform vital functions or tasks. Thus, a cell can't maintain itself or contribute to the organism. This leads to loss of tissue function, and then loss of organ function.

Number two: the gain of pathological function. When bad proteins cannot be eliminated, they accumulate in the cell. This can cause a crowding problem, as we will see soon, and physically block the ability of a cell to function. Unfortunately, however, the biggest issue is that it is not uncommon for these maladapted proteins to become toxic. There is even a term for this- Proteotoxicity.

• •

"Many diseases, including Alzheimer's, Parkinson's and Huntington's disease, are linked to the accumulation of toxic misfiled proteins in aggregates and inclusions."[6]

"Impairment of this fundamental function results in intracellular accumulation of potentially toxic protein structures, culminating in the triggering of cell death."[7]

• •

As noted, the failure of proteins, by any means, ultimately leads to cell failure and cell death or senescence.

We find then, that there is a balance between the rate of protein damage and the rate of clean up. When a cell is young, the damage is low and the ability to repair it is high. With age however, this gets reversed. The damage rises and the ability to repair it, or eliminate it, falls.

When enough damage accumulates, the cell is forced to either commit suicide, i.e., apoptosis, or become senescent. As we have learned, neither of these outcomes is beneficial. As more and more cells fall victim to failure, the organ fails as well.

Thus, "a progressive deterioration in the ability of cells to preserve the stability of their proteome occurs with age and contributes to the functional loss characteristic of old organisms."[5]

• •

"Failure to maintain protein homeostasis is associated with aggregation and cell death, and underlies a growing list of pathologies including neurodegenerative diseases, aging and cancer."[6]

"Especially during aging, a reduction in anti-oxidant defense mechanisms leads to an increased formation in free radical oxygen species and consequently results in a damage of proteins, including mitochondrial and synaptic ones. Even those proteins involved in repair and protein clearance via the ubiquitin proteasome and lysosomal system are subject to damage and show a reduced function."[8]

"Dysfunction of the quality control mechanisms and intracellular accumulation of abnormal proteins in the form of protein inclusions and aggregates occur in almost all tissues of an aged organism."[5]

"During aging, mitochondrial defects are increasingly occurring and resulting in the formation of ROS and increased protein oxidation. In addition, anti oxidation defense mechanisms are reduced, with defective protein repair and UPS dysfunction."[8]

• •

At this point in time, there is a significant base of knowledge concerning proteins and their extensive protective and repair devices. Unfortunately, there still isn't that much information about how to reverse the degradation that occurs.

Preventing the damage is the best strategy at the moment. Reducing the effect from ROS and free radicals, for example, are especially important.

In addition to this, there is some nascent evidence that we can upregulate the transcription of chaperones. Two types of evidence support the idea that this may be helpful. First, chaperone induction in single-cell and multi-cell organisms leads to increased longevity. Secondly, in centenarians, the ability to upregulate these proteins remains intact with their advanced age.[5] Therefore, the ability to maintain chaperones is clearly within human reach, we just need to figure out the details.

How do we increase our declining levels of chaperones? Interestingly, caloric restriction, a strategy known to improve lifespan in general, has also been shown to restore chaperone levels in aged tissues. Further, whereas it has not yet been studied, I would argue that the caloric restriction mimetics may also improve chaperone levels.

We now turn to the ultimate recycling program. As we have noted earlier, all things great and small can malfunction. Not only do DNA and proteins malfunction, entire organelles fail with time. As nutrients and the building blocks of cells are not unlimited in supply, the cells have evolved complex systems for recycling. Therefore, the cell tracks and then targets proteins, protein complexes, lipids and organelles that are suboptimal, separates them from the others, and consequently dismantles them into smaller components.

This is called autophagy, which literally means 'eating oneself.' What it really is, is a catabolic pathway that promotes the degradation and recycling of cellular components. Essentially, once identified and sequestered, the failing target is delivered to organelles called lysosomes. These small sacs, or vesicles, engulf the cargo and exposes them to dissolving or proteolytic enzymes.

The relevance of this process is determined by the length of life of a particular cell, as well as its ability to divide. If a cell is short-lived, the process isn't very important. The individual organelles don't need to get recycled, because soon enough the entire cell is going to get replaced. For long-lived, non-dividing cells, however this process is key to survival.

• •

> *Autophagy is... "an evolutionarily conserved recycling pathway that maintains protein and organelle quality control."*[9]
>
> *"Autophagy plays a crucial role in the degradation of long-lived proteins and organelles. These properties make autophagy a crucial mechanism for maintaining tissue homeostasis during the aging process."*[10]

• •

There are three main types of autophagy, delineated by the target itself.

1) Microautophagy: literally, the eating of little pieces (of any type of cellular debris).

2) Macroautophagy: Bigger pieces. These chunks are engulfed by a sac or vesicle which then fuses with a lysosome (another sac containing degrading enzymes). The prime example is a dysfunctional mitochondria. This is also referred to as Mitophagy.

3) Chaperone-Mediated autophagy: This is usually a maladaptive or criminal protein who gets ratted out by its chaperone, and hand delivered into a lysosome.

The actual subtypes of autophagy aren't exactly that important, but I remain fascinated by the complexity of the mechanisms available to help us live long and well. Unfortunately, as has been true for every good system, this one becomes dysfunctional with increasing age.

• •

> *"Autophagy declines with age, and the impairment of autophagy contributes to neurodegeneration, insulin resistance, cardiac hypertrophy and dysfunction, and osteoarthritis."*[10]
>
> *"A plethora of evidence has linked compromised autophagy to development of age related disorders."*[9]

• •

It is not clear exactly which part of the autophagy process fails over time; it probably occurs at many of the steps. We do know, however, that this leads to the incomplete degradation of the cargo inside the lysosomes. With advancing age, the cell sees an accumulation of undegraded products that stick together and become something called lipofuscin. I refer to this as the kitchen drawer phenomena. Over time, clutter develops everywhere, even in the most controlled situations, and it aways brings to mind the kitchen drawer in everyone's home that holds the odds and ends. This drawer, over the course of 20 years or so becomes packed with the most random items that never seem to get thrown away. Eventually, this **Or the drawer to open** ▶ accumulation of cellular debris blocks the ability of the cell to function.

OK, so autophagy is important, and of course it declines with age. What is there to do to increase it?

Luckily, over the last several years we have come to appreciate that there are several things that can be done.

1.   **Caloric restriction:** Again, good to know, but really quite impractical. The good news is that caloric restriction mimetics can have a similar effect.

• •

> *"The effects of caloric restriction on macroautophagy induction are believed to be mediated by the activation of either of two energy sensors, AMPK and SIRT1."*[9]

• •

2.　　**mTOR inhibition:** The classic mTOR inhibitor, rapamycin, is known to promote autophagy as well as increase lifespan. Unfortunately at this point, the side effects from this medication outweigh the benefits.

3.　　**AMP Kinase activators:** There are several known substances in this category. The most well known of which is metformin. Also working at several other aging dilemmas, this agent has few downsides.[10]

4.　　**Sirtuin1:** This family of youth genes can also serve as autophagy regulators. Conveniently, these are activated by resveratrol and pterostilbene.

5.　　**Exercise:** I know, once again, I said there would be no emphasis on exercise, but I can't help but include it. Exercise induces autophagy in skeletal muscle.

So, this leads us to the take-home message of this chapter. With aging comes more cellular damage and less of an ability to repair it. But alas, the end of this story has yet to be written.

CHAPTER 8:

SECURITY SYSTEMS - THE IMMUNE SYSTEM

Following our now familiar factory analogy, the immune system acts as our security department to keep out the bad guys and maintain the status quo. Threats can come both from external and internal sources, and like any good security detail, the body has a full time, extensive staff that is continuously on patrol.

In general, this is a great thing. In fact, it is phenomenal. We live in an extremely dangerous environment filled with bacteria, viruses, parasites, prions, and toxins, not to mention guns, poisons, radiation, smoke and nuclear radiation.

The body is frequently, if not constantly, being attacked by pathogens, defined as any biological agent that can harm or bring disease to its host, i.e., you. To combat the threats, the body is equipped with a multitiered and multimodal system of defense. These range from physical barriers like the skin, to a complex set of cells that can identify, attack and then even store the memory of said attack, to improve the odds of victory in ensuing confrontations.

Whereas this is not a primer on immunology, we will review a few of the basics before plunging into the *what goes wrong* conversation. For now, rest assured that just like in our factory model, the big security dudes that are supposed to guard you, can turn against the company and bring it down in the end.

The following discussion will review the basics of this system, then its dysfunction and consequent effects on aging can be better understood. Please bear with me if this seems either too complicated or too simplistic.

I can't make everyone happy all the time!

The immune system can be broken down into many different categories, but the most basic division separates the innate from the adaptive system. The innate system is the first line of defense, and it is speedy and efficient. It can be thought of as the first responders in an actual emergency, functioning much like a paramedic or an emergency room. The system is non-specific in that it responds to every situation as well as it can, but it is restricted to basic treatments. For example, the paramedic can place an IV and perhaps give a medication or two, but your brain surgery is going to have to wait for the specialist.

The most obvious component of our innate system is our integument (skin) and the mucous membranes that separate us from our environment. Our skin is pretty impressive and does an incredible job of protecting us. The real day to day threats actually attack us through the openings in our integument that cannot be sealed off as effectively. Our lungs, for example, are a prime target as we continuously breath in foreign substances. Because of this, coughing and sneezing have developed to mechanically remove any irritants from the respiratory tract. Tiny cilia, or little hairs, exist as well that are constantly in motion, pushing any foreign substances up and out of the lungs.

In addition, there are chemicals that prevent substances in our lungs from breaching our defenses and causing infections.

Similar repellant and protective systems are in fact at work all over the body. Antibacterials exist in our saliva, tears and even breast milk. The acid in our stomach kills undesirable bacteria that we may have swallowed. Meanwhile, on a friendlier note, we allow other, helpful bacteria to coexist all over our bodies to fend off the evil pathogens.

Still examining the innate system, we turn to the leukocytes or white blood cells. These cells are produced in our bone marrow, and continuously roam around, seeking out pathogens. There are innumerable types of white cells, but the most important include the neutrophils and the macrophages. As a group, these cells first identify and then collaborate to extinguish most threats. Both of these cell types fall into a classification called phagocytes, which are reminiscent of the game Pac-man. The cells track down and find pathogens, and then ingest and destroy them.

They even beep as they go too! ▶

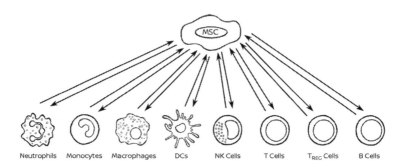

Neutrophils   Monocytes   Macrophages   DCs   NK Cells   T Cells   T_{REG} Cells   B Cells

Neutrophils are the most abundant of this population, making up about 60 to 70% of the circulating white blood cells. During an acute bacterial infection, these cells either stumble upon the crime scene independently or they respond to chemical help signals. Distressed cells release cytokines as an emergency signal, and neutrophils and other first responders migrate to the site. Referred to as chemotaxis, signals from the infected site travel all over the body; thus the response and the inflammatory reaction tends to be global, not just localized. So, in our analogy of first responders, calling for neutrophils is like calling the ambulance. If for fun, or simply curiosity, you examined a glob of yellowish, white pus under a microscope, you would see mostly neutrophils.

I'm sure there's an app for that ▶

In terms of numbers, a standard human produces about 10^{11} neutrophils a day and they live between five and ninety hours. This is truly rapid cell turnover that isn't problematic for the body when you are young; your neutrophils live by the play hard and die young motto. As we all know too well, however, this lifestyle becomes more of a challenge with advancing age.

Then the motto becomes take it easy and try not to die ▶

Continuing on, if you have too few neutrophils, you are neutropenic.

This can be a side effect of chemotherapy, a sign of cancer or disease, or just old age. Common sense tells us it is just not good to be neutropenic, as the risk of uncontrolled infection can skyrocket.

Interestingly, neutrophils are much like people in their dietary choices; not the vegetarians or the health nuts, just the normal standard person. Presented with a tasty molecule of glucose (or fructose, sucrose or honey) versus a succulent, enticing bacteria, the phagocyte will choose the sugar every time. Therefore, neutrophils are less effective in high glucose environments, electing to consume the glucose instead of the pathogen. This is one of the reasons that diabetics get terrible infections.

Macrophages (i.e., big eaters, by Greek roots) meanwhile, tend to hang out in the tissues and not circulate as much. They congregate several days after the initiating event, and replace the neutrophils as the predominant cell type. These versatile cells produce enzymes, proteins and regulatory factors that are crucial to localizing the infection and walling off the pathogen. These cells also emit very powerful inflammatory factors, including Interleukin-1(IL-1), IL-6, and Tumor necrosis Factor-α.

Macrophages also act as waste engineers once the area has been secured. It rids the body of worn out cells and unwanted debris, and can even dispose of aged neutrophils. Compared to neutrophils, macrophages live a bit longer, somewhere between four to fifteen days. This is still a very limited lifespan however, and the supply must be continuously replenished.

Of note, macrophages come in two main varieties. M1's are the Killer macrophages; they secrete the inflammatory cytokines and consume pathogens. These inflammatory factors, including innumerable types of interleukins, become a huge problem with aging.

M2's, by contrast, are considered 'repair' cells. They assist in the reconstruction of tissue following an event, especially wound healing and tissue mending.

As smart as the body is, however, frequently the enemy is even smarter; Tuberculosis (TB) is one such example. The pathogen, *Mycobacterium tuberculosis*, actually lives inside of the macrophage after invading the body through the lungs. In fact, this white cell becomes its hideout, effectively protecting itself from other modes of attack. This strategy turns out to be pretty effective as TB has proven difficult to eradicate as a disease.

Mast cells, a less numerous subtype of leukocytes, reside in connective tissue and mucus membranes. They play a role in wound healing, blood vessels production (angiogenesis), and protection of the blood-brain barrier. Importantly, these cells contain granules or inclusions that release histamine and heparin when activated. Heparin is an anticoagulant that blocks clotting and thus allows more blood to flow to the area. Histamine is responsible for dilating blood vessels which also brings more blood to the effected area, and assists with inflammatory functions.

In reality, though, histamine is quite annoying. We have all experienced it. It is the cause of itching (pruritus), simple allergies and even anaphylaxis (a life-threatening allergy), for which bug bites are a classic example. A microscopic bite leads to pain, redness and an incredible amount of itching. We slather on the calamine lotion, but yet we still itch and itch. Thus, histamine blockers, most commonly diphenhydramine or benadryl (the brand name), are one of the most commonly used over the counter medications.

No one likes to itch! ▶

Basophils and eosinophils are less interesting, with the caveat that clearly I'm not an immunologist. I'm sure innumerable folks have dedicated their lives to these little cells, but still, they are less than exciting. They are just another component of the immune system, but are far less in number. They are more active in parasitic infections, and release a plethora of cytokines and other mediators of inflammation.

Natural killer cells, the last cells of the innate immune system, do not attack foreign invaders or pathogens. These cells actually destroy the bodies own cells that have gone astray. Considered compromised host cells, these can be cells that are either infected with viruses or they are cancer cells. Either way, natural killer cells show no mercy. If a human cell has gone bad, it gets taken out before it negatively affects some other cell.

The adaptive immune system is the second component in the defensive battle, and it retains the memory of the enemy. In other words, it allows the host (us) to have an improved response if there is a second or third attack; this is how immunization works. Using a compliment of several cell types, this system is able to recognize very specific foreign attackers once they have been seen once, and then store this information.

The cells in this system are called lymphocytes, and are broken down mostly into B cells and T cells.

T cells: These cells originate in the bone marrow, but they mature in the thymus. You probably have never heard of the thymus, but it's a small organ that sits above the heart. It is much larger in kids and can be visualized on a chest X-ray; it usually disappears in adults so you don't ever hear about it. Regardless, you carry between 25 million to one billion different T cells in your body. Each has a unique receptor that can identify only one antigen. You theoretically have at least one T cell for every pathogen that you have already been exposed to.

Killer T cells: These awesomely named cells find and destroy infected human cells that have been turned into virus production centers. T cells can identify a bad host cell by virtue of viral pieces that aren't completely engulfed, and thus they protrude from the cell. When the Killer T cell attaches to the infected cell, it releases a protein called perforin that perforates the cell, and injects cytotoxins. Thus, the bad cell is eradicated. Remnants of the destroyed cells are then cleaned up by macrophages. Of note, these are also called CD8 cells.

Helper T cell: These cells don't make toxins or fight invaders themselves, instead, they serve as coordinators. They send out cytokines or chemical messengers to direct the other pieces of the immune system. (CD4 cells)

B cells: These cells are also made in the bone marrow and are responsible for producing very specialized proteins called antibodies. A discussion of this topic could go on for pages and pages, so I'm going to keep this extremely simple.

Antibodies are Y shaped proteins that come in a variety of configurations (different numbers of Y's stuck together) and their job is to identify and adhere to specific pathogens. Once the invader is labeled, it can be disposed of.

The antibody subtypes differ by both body location and how many are attached to each other. IgG is a single Y shape, and is the most common antibody type there is. It is also the only one that can cross from mother to fetus in utero. IgA, on the other hand, is found in mucosal areas, like the GI tract, respiratory tract and the urogenital tract, and is also found in saliva, tears, and breast milk. Physically, IgA is a dimer, meaning there are two Y shaped pieces connected at the ends.

To round out the discussion, IgE, also a single Y, releases histamine from mast cells and basophils. It also protects against parasitic worms. There are others, like IgM and IgD, but we don't really need to know this.

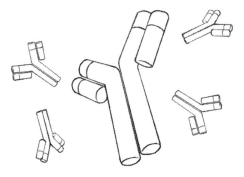

Enough of the primer on immunology... How does all this effect aging?

There are 3 main issues central to aging in the immunology sphere.

1. The body gets put in a chronic state of inflammation that becomes responsible for innumerable, terrible disease states of aging.
2. The risk of infection rises.
3. There is an increase in cancers, especially in the cells that originate from bone marrow.

The biggest issue is inflammation. So let's tackle it first.

• •

"Levels of inflammatory mediators typically increase with age even in the absence of acute infection or other physiological stress."[1]

"The aging process is a chronic smoldering oxidative and inflammatory stress that leads to the damage of cellular components, including proteins, lipids, and DNA, contributing to the age-related decline of physiological functions."[1]

• •

Inflammation, as a process, is part of the complex response to pathogens. It's one of the first steps in fighting any disturbance, and thus serves to set the immune system in the right direction. This response involves an increase in blood flow, with an influx of white blood cells, innumerable cellular mediators and cytokines.

The classic signs of inflammation are pain, redness, swelling and increased temperature, which make a lot of sense. When the body perceives an infection, it sends in the cavalry. The process begins with an increased blood flow so that the necessary elements can get to the site. This accounts for the visible redness, and the increase in temperature. These blood vessels also become more permeable, meaning leaky, and the specialized mediators jump out of the vasculature and into the infected site. Fluids leak out as well, and this leads to the swelling. If this becomes too severe, it impinges or squishes nerves, and this can cause pain.

• •

Of note, the application of a cold compress causes the blood vessels to tighten, and thus you get less swelling. A heating pad, meanwhile, increases blood flow which causes more swelling, but also an influx of cellular mediators.

• •

The goal of the system, of course, is to eradicate the disease, clean out the necrotic or dead tissue, and then restore function. As an acute mechanism, this system works quite well. Healthy folks are generally able to stave off most serious infections.

The body, however, as we have established, doesn't always know when enough is enough. Unfortunately, an acute inflammation is often followed by a chronic inflammation. This chronic state manifests as a nagging, unending agony, the specifics of which depend on the tissue effected.

As well, chronic inflammation can begin without an obvious inciting factor, and simply reek a slow, merciless havoc on the body. Aging is one of these situations. Chronic low grade inflammation is so frequently associated with aging in fact that there is a name for it: 'Inflammaging.' Recognized as a corner stone in the aging process around 2000, study after study has demonstrated the significant degree of damage that accrues over time. From obesity, diabetes, pulmonary and metabolic diseases, to atherosclerosis and neural degeneration, chronic inflammation plays a tremendous role.

We know that inflammation gets worse with age because we can actually measure it. In fact, we can quantify the degree of both acute and chronic inflammation by looking at specific markers in the blood. There are a zillion potential things to measure, so researchers are trying to narrow it down.

Presently, the known factors that are highly correlated to aging are the following: Interleukin-1, Interleukin-6, Interleukin-18, C-reactive protein (CRP), Tumor Necrosis Factor-alpha (TNF-α), serum Amyloid, Soluble vascular cell adhesion molecule-1 (sVCAM-1), and Monocyte chemoattractant protein-1(MCP-1).

With age, most, if not all of the inflammatory cytokines increase. In a study trying to figure out which ones were most correlated with age and mortality, IL-6 and (ultra sensitive) CRP levels had the most robust association with time of survival, independent of cause of death. IL-10 and IL-1β were highly associated with all forms of death except cardiovascular disease. Interestingly, in those 80 years or older, a low IL-6 could predict, all by itself, if an 80 year old would live 3 more years.[2]

So, why does this occur? Why is it that these once useful cytokines are now the flag bearers of doom? And why are they out of control?

The increase of these cytokines actually comes from several sources. For one, we need to consider our aging cells. The process of a cell becoming senescent will be addressed in the next chapter, but suffice it to say that as the longer-lived cells get old, they do not fare very well. Using our factory analogy, the older cell resembles the near to retirement employee. They sort of do their job, but mostly they just complain and irritate anyone around them. In a similar fashion, the senescent cell emits inflammatory cytokines, thus eliciting an inflammatory response both locally and systemically. Again, this will be addressed more later, but the cells are called SASPs or have Senescence-Associated Secretory Phenotypes. Regardless, as we age, we accumulate more and more senescent cells, and the inflammatory system rages out of control.

Senescent cells, however, are not the only producers of inflammatory factors. As people age, another occurrence is the accumulation of increasing fat stores, especially in the abdominal area. All fat produces and releases inflammatory cytokines, especially IL-6. Visceral or abdominal fat produces at least three times the amount from that of fat stored elsewhere. As well, fat houses macrophages that we know also secrete inflammatory factors. Therefore, the abdominal tire syndrome that we see in middle age not only looks unattractive, but also accelerates the aging process.

Glucose is also problematic. Glucose binds with proteins, DNA and lipids to form a complex called an AGE or an Advanced Glycation Endpoint that inflicts irreparable damage all over the body. Regardless, one of the side products of AGEs is the production of more inflammatory factors.

Another thing we need to address is the actual inflammatory tree. It's actually an upside down tree, in that there are a few mediators at the top, but these activate a zillion more inflammatory factors in a downward, domino effect.

Tumor necrosis Factor (TNF) and Nuclear Factor kappa-Beta (NF-$\kappa\beta$) sit at the top of this tree. TNF activates the Nuclear factor, which then travels into the cell's nucleus. This mediator then turns on over 400 genes that are involved in the inflammatory pathway. Therefore, this system has earned a few minutes of our time.

TNF senses the environment and gets activated by insults to the cells. These can come in the form of undesirable bacteria, viruses, environmental pollutants, physical or mechanical stress, high glucose environments, UV radiation… the list is endless. The information is then transmitted to NF-$\kappa\beta$ and the cascade begins.

This cascade, unfortunately, leads to aging. The good news is that there are innumerable things we can do to curb this phenomena.

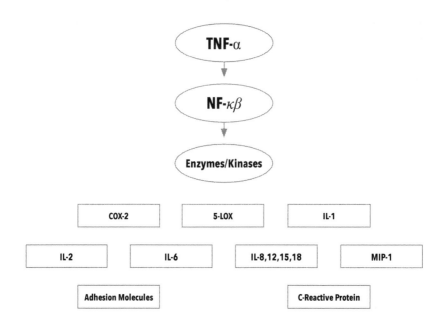

• •

"Inflammaging is a highly significant risk factor for both morbidity and mortality in elderly people, as most if not all age-related diseases share an inflammatory pathogenesis."[3]

• •

The second major complication of an aging immune system is the inability to fight off disease; in fact, the functionality of all types of immunity declines. For one, the body becomes unable to keep up with the demand for the high cell turnover; there just aren't enough cells to patrol the body. This problem originates from a declining stem cell population in the bone marrow, which is yet another unfortunate hallmark of aging.

• •

"One of the main features in human aging is the loss of adult stem cell homeostasis."[4]

• •

As well, the cells that do exist do not function as effectively. Macrophages become less aggressive, the killer cells rethink their philosophy, B cells become less competent, and as a result, the body loses the ability to create functional antibodies. Not only does this add to the declining immune system as a whole, it prevents the body from creating antibodies in response to vaccines. Therefore, while a child or healthy adult is protected by a vaccine, an older person may not be. Macrophages, in addition, become less effective, and as a last insult, and with significantly advanced age, the skin becomes less able to ward off even the most seemingly benign pathogens.

The last problem with the aging immune system is the propensity to develop bone marrow-based cancers. As the stem cells decline in number and function, they tend to produce abnormal cells. These issues result in a very high incidence of malignancies. Further, it is also known that the elevated inflammatory state can contribute to cancer as well.

• •

> *"It is well understood that proinflammatory states are linked to tumor production."*[5]

> *"Advanced age is associated with a declining ability to mount satisfactory immune responses resulting in increased infection susceptibility and diminished vaccine-elicited immune responses. Paradoxically, aged individuals also have a reduced ability to resolve certain types of inflammation leading to chronic, low grade inflammatory responses and the development of inflammation-associated comorbidities, such as cardiovascular disease, autoimmunity, and malignancy."*[6]

• •

It is therefore obvious that our once helpful immune system loses control over time.

Scientists, physicians and drug companies are well aware of the high potential for anti-inflammatories. As such, they account for a huge percentage of both the over the counter and behind the counter drug sales.

There are innumerable anti-inflammatories that come to us both by way of unadulterated natural substances, modified natural substances, and then completely lab-derived substances. Whereas I am in no way biased in considering natural versus not so natural products, there does seem to be a correlation with man-made or man-engineered substances and side effects.

In the anti-inflammatory category, without a doubt, the most powerful medications are steroids. More specifically, glucocorticoids are steroids that are used, usually, in acute and dramatic situations where the inflammatory reaction can be life threatening, painful, or just very serious. A good example might be a severe asthma attack, where the ability to breath is put at risk. Additionally, gout, painful osteoarthritic joints and Crohn's disease exacerbations are good examples. Specific medications in this division include cortisol, cortisone, prednisone, dexamethasone, beclometasone and many others.

The onset and efficacy of these meds is impressive. Almost immediately, people tend to feel better as their symptoms subside. Unfortunately, the side effect profile of steroids is terrible: immunodeficiency, hyperglycemia, skin fragility, easy bruising, osteoporosis, obesity, adrenal insufficiency, muscle breakdown, growth failure, glaucoma, cataract formation....the list goes on and on.

Clearly, a short-term course of steroids for an emergent issue can be acceptable, but the long term use for the purposes of anti-aging would not be indicated. You would die or dwindle from side effects before you had the chance to get old.

COX-2 inhibitors belong to a group of medications called non-steroidal anti-inflammatory drugs (or NSAIDS) that directly targets COX-2, an enzyme responsible for pain and inflammation. Synthesis of COX-2 is upregulated by the cytokines IL-1 and TNF-α, and specific inhibitors of COX-2 have been particularly useful in treating the pain component associated with rheumatoid arthritis or osteoarthritis.

One of the most popular of these drugs is Celecoxib (Celebrex) which was introduced onto the market in 1999. At one time there were several of these medications available, including Rofecoxib (Vioxx) and Valdecoxib (Bextra). These drugs were remarkably popular; sales of Celebrex alone reached 3.1 billion dollars in 2001. As compared to other NSAIDS, especially naproxen or ibuprofen, they were found to have fewer GI side effects. Sadly, few things are ever as good as they seem. It was soon determined that Vioxx and some of the other COX-2 inhibitors substantially increased the risk of myocardial infarctions (heart attacks). Thus, a warning was released in 2002 concerning the increased risk of cardiovascular events (stroke and heart attacks) with these medications. At the present, Celebrex is one of the few still available.

In the over the counter category, there is ibuprofen and naproxen. Ibuprofen was discovered in 1961, marketed in the United States in 1974 and became an over the counter medication in 1984. The drug has potential gastrointestinal side effects and is associated with increased risk of cardiovascular disease at high doses.

• •

Rumor has it that ibuprofen was first tested on a hangover by its discoverer, Stewart Adams.

• •

Naproxen, meanwhile, has an intermediate risk of gastric ulceration as compared to ibuprofen, but has the least overall cardiovascular risk. It was originally available by prescription in the US in 1976, but became available over the counter in 1994.

My absolute favorite anti-inflammatory however, is all natural and has been around for thousands of years. In fact, it is one of my all time favorite substances. When people say something is so amazing it can cure cancer, usually they are kidding. Here, it's true.

Curcumin can actually help prevent cancer.

It's almost time for to discuss all of all the agents that can stop all the doom and gloom!

CHAPTER 9:

THE WORKER BEES - CHALLENGES OF THE CELL

In our continuing factory analogy, we now turn to the actual worker bees, which for us are our individual cells. Our bodies are essentially composed of cells, which makes this a very important topic.

Some of the employees at our plant are young and enthusiastic, some are overweight and middle-aged, while others are old and mercilessly grumpy. There are a few college kids that work for a few months to make money over the summer, while some folks are as old as the bricks in the building itself. Amazingly enough, the cells in our bodies embody many, if not all, of these same characteristics.

So, despite what I have been implying thus far, not all cells are the same. Clearly, a brain cell is different from a red blood cell. One is stationary and transmits information; the other is constantly moving, transporting oxygen and carbon dioxide throughout the body. Clearly, the functions of the cells are quite varied. But more importantly, at least for this chapter, the longevity and thus the associated challenges that each type of cell faces, is vastly different.

Each red blood cell in your body is only going to live for a few months, three to four at best. This is why you can donate blood. Within a few months, your red cell population returns to normal as cell production ramps up to replace the missing cells. The average brain cell, however, is going to live years, if not your entire lifespan. As such, I wouldn't donate too many brain cells. As you may have guessed, from the very short-lived cell to the very long-lived cell, the rate-limiting factors for each are not the same.

First, let's figure out which cells are which.

Some of our cells are turned over incredibly rapidly, even much faster than red blood cells. Leukocytes, for example, last somewhere between 5 to 60 hours as we mentioned in the last chapter.

The cells lining your gastrointestinal system get turned over every 1 to 5 days. Since our stomachs contain strong acids and enzymes, it would not be unexpected that the cells containing these acids get macerated regularly and need to be replaced. You actually turn over cells so rapidly throughout your entire GI tract that even if you didn't eat much of anything, you still accumulate a sizable pile of refuse in your gut. For this reason, even if you haven't consumed anything, you'll still need to poop.

The cells on the tip of your tongue, meanwhile, turn over in about 10 days. You probably already sort of know this, especially if you have burned your tongue. It takes about that long for your mouth to feel normal again. The skin epidermis, or outer layer, takes between 10 to 30 days. You may be aware of this as well; it takes about that long to repair sunburned skin.

In the slightly longer category, sperm replacement takes about 2 months.

It's too easy to make jokes here... I'll leave it alone!

Bone cell turnover takes about 3 months. As mentioned earlier, red cells live about 4 months. This seems like a long time by comparison, but the body makes about 100 million new red blood cells every minute. This is because the total number of circulating red blood cells, 3×10^{13} is huge. Thus, by comparison the turnover is moderate. You also make 10^{11} neutrophils per day. In essence, you have very active bone marrow.

Moving onto the slower categories, many tissues get replaced that we once thought were rather permanent. One such example are the cells that constitute your heart muscle. As luck would have it, these get replaced, although pretty slowly, at a rate of 0.5 to 10% per year. So, alas, there is a cure for the broken heart. But as we all already know... the recovery from a broken heart is very slow.

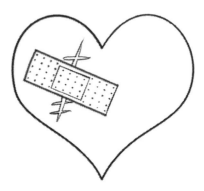

Most of the skeleton gets turned over at the rate of 10% per year. Your ear bones, however, generally don't get turned over at all; these are with you your entire life.

Adipose, or fat cells, are similar to bone and turn over at a rate of 8% per year.

So if someone is on your last nerve, you really do have a problem. On the farthest end of the timing spectrum, most nerve cells tend to last a lifetime.

The cells that make up the lens in the eye are also permanent.

• •

Random but cool info: Hair grows about 1 cm per month. Fingernails grow about 0.3 cm per month.

• •

Just for fun, we are going to take a closer look at some of the more important tissues in your body.

Neurons

Most neurons, i.e. nerve cells in the brain and spinal cord, are permanent. In fact, less than 1% of olfactory nerves (nerves that are responsible for smelling) or cerebral cortex (thinking) neurons turn over within a century. These are present when you are an infant, and last as long as they can without replacement. This is why, at the present time, if you sever your spinal cord and all the nerves with it, you are permanently paralyzed. Scientists are working hard to try to fix this, but at the moment, there is no cure for such severe nerve damage.

There is, however, a subpopulation of neurons in the hippocampus, specifically the dentate gyrus, that do turnover. Why this area of the brain? The dentate gyrus is thought to contribute to the formation of new, episodic memories and the spontaneous exploration of novel environments. Therefore, the creation of new nerves may allow the formation of new thoughts and memories.

Anyway, of this dentate gyrus hippocampal population, 35% of the nerve cells are constantly getting exchanged. Despite being a very small and select area of the brain, it turns out that this is not trivial. The body creates about 700 of these new neurons in the hippocampus every day. This is a lot of cells. As a result, this population has an annual turnover of 1.75%. Of note, the newly created cells actually have a shorter lifespan, about 7.1 years, which is 10X shorter than the permanent cells.[1]

As well in the brain, the non-neuronal or support cells, mostly astrocytes and microglia, turn over at a rate of 3.5% per year. This isn't as bad as not turning over at all, but this low number translates into more problems for the permanent cells. It mean that the environmental niche that supports the neurons is going to fail over time, depriving them of the necessary nutrients and the healthy environment that supports their functions. This is yet another reason that the brain does not do as well as the other parts of the body with the onset of advanced age.

In addition to the slow, if not nonexistent, cell turnover in the central nervous system, the brain faces many other hurdles. If you think about it, our neurons are more challenged than most cells. They are in an odd position in that they are sprinting a marathon, for years on end.

Brain cells have an extremely high metabolic rate; they utilize excessive amounts of glucose and oxygen. High oxygen consumption leads to an increase in free radical production, and free radicals love to attack and destroy lipids (as well as DNA and proteins). The brain has a very high concentration of lipids and as such, is a prime target for peroxidation attack. The brain, thus, suffers from its own doing.

It makes sense then, that over time, there is an absolute and constant loss of neurons. By the age of eighty, there is a 10-15% decrease in brain weight, and a 20% reduction in cerebral blood flow as a consequence. Therefore, it is easy to understand why there is a decline in neurologic function. Frequently, this is when many people begin to understand that aging is real. Many people don't notice their enlarged girths, their gray hair or even their increasing fatigue. But start losing your mind, and all of a sudden, aging becomes real.

Anyway, over time, there is known memory loss, progressive hearing loss, reduced amount, speed and dexterity of motor activity, reduced muscular power, and impaired stance, posture and gait.[2] At this point, there is little to nothing that can be done to salvage the situation. Luckily, you are reading this now, hopefully before you have begun losing your marbles. Therefore, with additional luck, we can prevent or delay the onset of some or all of these neurological issues.

Bone[3]

The skeleton is more user-friendly than the brain and its neurons. It is staffed with an enthusiastic team of workers that are constantly remodeling. Some of these employees work demolition; taking the bone apart and sending the pieces to the recycling department; these are the osteoclasts. Other workers, perhaps the more creative ones, follow behind and rebuild; these are the osteoblasts, (blast for build). Thus, the skeleton is constantly being remodeled and repaired. This is why broken bones heal themselves over time.

You can't fix your brain, but healing a broken tibia is a piece of cake!

Under normal circumstances, this process is well balanced. With advancing age, of course, the balance is lost. More bone gets destroyed than created, and the skeleton loses strength and integrity. One might say that the remodeling design becomes more 'modern' or stark over time. The bone density decreases, the collagen infrastructure weakens, and the mineralization can decline as well. As a result, the bone strength and resilience deteriorates.

Therefore, the older you get, the more likely you are to break a bone, and the longer it takes to heal. Unfortunately for women, especially when postmenopausal, the loss of bone occurs at an even more accelerated rate.

This deficiency in building with advancing age is thought to be due to a loss in the number of osteoblasts. These cells arise from mesenchymal stem cells whose function also declines with age. There are in fact many reasons the bone fails with age, but this is thought to be the most important.

Regardless, there is a deficiency in the cells that you require, and an increase in ones that you do not.

The take-home message in all of this is simple: you need a constant supply of new, somewhat short-lived cells that are produced by very long-lived, stem cells.

Of note, different bones and bone cells age at different rates; turnover times vary widely from bone to bone.

Fat[1]

The fat cell is an annoying thing. We have to have some, but we certainly don't want to have many. Further, they seem to be located in places we really don't want them. From a personnel perspective, I picture them as middle management. They are necessary, but a little irritating. As well, they seem to last for years, just hanging out and collecting their paychecks.

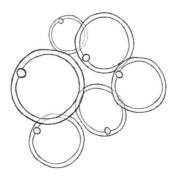

Of course, despite my sarcasm, fat cells are important. Humans evolved a long time ago when calories were not as easy to come by, and the storage of energy for the lean times was quite necessary. Therefore, our bodies developed a system to be able to store energy in the form of fat, and then mobilize it when needed. Unfortunately, or not, in today's world, very few of us are starving. Therefore, we have ample fat and cells to store it in.

Based on your environment when you are young, as well as genetics, the body has to make some permanent choices. One of these is how many fat cells to have. It is decided, in fact, by the age of twenty, roughly, exactly how many fat cells the body needs. Following this decision, that number does not change. The actual number of fat cells does however, vary tremendously from person to person. The obese kid is going to go into adulthood having way more fat cells than a skinny kid. How exactly this occurs is unknown, but the obese kid is never going to decrease their number of fat cells. They can decrease the volume of fat in each cell, but not the number of cells. The only way to actually decrease the number of fat cells is to have them sucked out by a plastic surgeon.

So, as we gain and lose fat over time, each individual cell is simply getting more or less full, either fluffy or flat. Even after extreme loss after bariatric surgery, the cells get smaller, but they certainly don't go away.

This set number of cells, however, does get turned over. Interestingly, between 8 to 10% of the cells get replaced yearly, which is completely independent of how many you have in the first place.

Pancreas[5]

The pancreas is an important organ to consider as it is the sole producer of insulin. Production of insulin occurs in beta-islet cells, and the failure to do so causes diabetes - a very serious, life-limiting condition.

Insulin is necessary to transport glucose into any and all cells. It acts as the key to the cell, or as the doorman. Without insulin, all cells would starve even while the circulation and extracellular tissues are awash in glucose. Therefore, failure to produce insulin causes systemic failure.

Once it was thought that the beta-islet cell population could respond to requirements and make more cells; and it does, sort of. Like fat cells, beta cells can alter their number up until the age of 20, when about 97% of the cell population is established. The most active beta cell turnover occurs at the age of 5, and then levels off. After the age of 20, each individual cell just has to try a little harder. Thus, these cells aren't as long-lived as nerve cells, but still have to survive a very long time under stressful conditions. By the time humans get older and fatter and the insulin requirement rises, the beta cells do the best they can until they run out of steam. Then, diabetes kicks in.

The point here is that tissues last for different lengths of time, and that each individual tissue or cell has its own challenges. For purposes of simplicity, cells fall into the following categories:

1. **Live hard and die fast:** These cells must get replaced very quickly, with no break in the production for as long as you live. These are the assembly line workers; low wage, fast turnover. They have a low commitment to the factory, but are essential regardless.

2. **Goldilocks cells:** Not too long, not too short. These are like middle management; they give you years of service, but ultimately they need to move on. Replacement is slow, but necessary.

3. **Extremely long-lived:** These are the permanent employees; they have been with the factory since the doors opened. They are sage, non-replaceable and we suffer as organisms when they suffer. They will either die in the line of service, or turn into bitter old men that ultimately become toxic.

All of these cell types are important for us, and they all face different challenges over time. Let's look at the longest of these cell types first.

To begin with, these cells are stationary; they aren't going anywhere. Thus, these cells require a constant and secure delivery system with enough raw materials to be fully functional. This requires an intact circulatory system complete with a good heart, good oxygen delivery, and appropriate nutrients.

Picture grandma getting her groceries delivered right from the store!

These cells are also engaged in a lifetime battle with oxidative and free radical stress that inflicts continuous damage. Even with all of the repair and quality control systems functioning around the clock, damage still accrues. Errors arise in the DNA and the proteins and over time, the cells suffer.

The other problem with long-lived cells is garbage. This is going to get more detailed in the next chapter, but for now it's important to note that as a cell gets older, they get filled up with cellular waste. Called lipofuscin, the pile gets so unruly that cellular functions get disturbed.

Thus, over time, there is a decline in the robustness of the cell and an increased risk of death. This isn't good when there is no cell coming to replace it.

The other key category of long-lived cells are the stem cells. In some ways they are the same as our long-lived nerve cells. They are not ambulatory, and they require a specialized, niche environment, and a delivery system for nutrients. There are also differences, however, as stem cells have the ability to hibernate when they are not needed.

It's a pretty cool and effective trick!

What exactly are stem cells?

• •

"In essence, stem cells are undifferentiated, long-lived cells that are unique in their abilities to produce differentiated daughter cells and to retain their stem cell identity by self renewal."[6]

• •

Stem cells can do essentially two major things. One, they produce an almost endless supply of new cells, that can then differentiate into the required, specific cells. Two, they must protect themselves from the pressures of time.

This form of cellular protection comes in several flavors. For starters, the cells have the capacity to hibernate or become quiescent when they are not needed. Much like a wintering bear, the stem cell alters its metabolism, turns off all major energy-requiring systems and becomes dormant until its services are required. Scientists believe this process evolved to protect the cell from the stresses that age most cells.

While this is occurring, the mitochondria actually change shape, and produce a lot less energy. As a result, fewer free radicals are generated and the DNA is thought to be somewhat protected. When it's time to activate a stem cell, one of the first steps is turning on the mitochondria; a cell needs energy first and foremost.

• •

Of note, a shortage of nicotinamide with advancing age (as we mentioned earlier) is thought to be rate limiting in activating stem cells.[7]

• •

In the scientific lingo, stem cell quiescence protects them from functional exhaustion and acts as a cellular mechanism to delay mutations leading to cancer.

This process isn't limited to animals; interestingly, dormant plant seeds are about the same. Seeds shut down until the right conditions present themselves, and then they germinate.

• •

"Adult stem cells are endowed with the remarkable ability to make, maintain, and repair tissues. As such, they are tasked with maintaining tissue homeostasis throughout the lifetime of the organism. In order for them to fulfill this responsibility, SC's are kept in a quiescent state in between their utilization. This reduces their exposure to metabolic and replicative stress, thereby preserving their genomic integrity."[8]

"Stem cell quiescence is an evolved adaptation to reduce metabolic byproducts, preserve genomic integrity, and ensure stem cell maintenance."[9]

• •

Another form of cellular protection is the enzyme telomerase. If you remember from the gene chapter, telomeres are long, non-coding sequences of base pairs at the tail ends of DNA that serve as protection caps. Overtime as the DNA is copied, the chain gets progressively shorter, and eventually it gets too short. When this occurs, the cell is no longer able to divide.

In case you forgot, this is really bad! ▶

Clearly as a stem cell, the inability to divide defeats its very purpose. Therefore, the cell produces something very special- telomerase. This enzyme is actually capable of adding base pairs back onto the DNA chain. In a way, telomerase can turn back time; at least on a cellular level.

Telomerase is absent or found at extremely low levels in most normal, somatic cells. Luckily, it is present in normal proliferating stem cells. Evidence for this comes from stem cells in the basal layer of the epidermis, human adult testis and ovaries. Unfortunately, but as per usual, good things decline over time and as such the quantity of telomerase drops with age.

We can fix this; don't worry! ▶

Like our bear in its winter cave, the stem cell resides in a specialized environment or niche. This micro-environment acts as physical protection and housing, provides a nourishing environment, and produces the chemical signals that communicate with the stem cell. Interestingly, the stem cell niche or nursery, lives in a state of relative hypoxia. The niches generally are less than 5% oxygen, which is significantly less than in the rest of us. In experimental conditions, increased amounts of oxygen are actually detrimental to stem cells. This specialized microenvironment is actually all about the neighborhood.

Location... Location... Location ▶

Once the stem cells are activated, they are phenomenal. The system allows for massive and repetitive regeneration, and can support all of the new cells that we have been referring to. The other thing to note is that within the bone marrow, the number of active stem cells can vary tremendously. Depending on need, there are is an ever-changing ratio of proliferating stem cells to the reserve of nonactive cells.

• •

Within this nursery, there are far more support cells than actual stem cells. For example, there are only about 2 to 5 hematopoietic stem cells per 10^5 total bone marrow cells.[10]

• •

So where are these niches? They are everywhere, as it turns out. In almost every body tissue, there is a localized cluster of stem cells. The largest stem cell collection resides in the bone marrow, but they are also in the liver, brain, fat, and intestine. Even hair follicles have stem cells.

Stem cells and aging

Stem cells, as we have seen, have developed fairly complex methods to stave off the effects of time. Unfortunately, these systems are not flawless. As such:

• •

> *"It is generally accepted that stem cell aging is the primary factor that drives the aging of tissues, and, importantly, underlies the aging of biological systems that are characterized by a high cellular turnover."*[10]

• •

So, what happens to stem cells with age?

1. The absolute number of viable stem cells diminish.

2. The differentiation potential in terms of the cell type able to be produced, and the number to be produced by stem cells declines. For example, older mesenchymal stem cells are less likely to become osteogenic (bone-building) or chondrogenic (cartilage-building). Instead, they turn into fat cells. (just what we need... more fat and less bone)

• •

> *"Age-dependent reduction in stem cell number or perturbed cell-cycle activity has been reported in skeletal muscle stem cells, neural stem cells and germline stem cells."*[11]

• •

3. The ability of stem cells to repair their own DNA fails. The DNA damage Response (DDR) normally seen in younger stem cells has a compromised capacity to repair.[12] As well, there is a significant decline in the cells telomerase activity.

4. Like any cell that has a long lifespan, there is concern over the ability to successfully produce proteins. Referred to as proteostasis or rather the homeostasis of protein production, it is the ability of a cell to synthesize, fold and turnover proteins. Defects in proteostasis leads to aberrant folding, toxic aggregation and the accumulation of damaged proteins that can lead to more cellular damage and tissue dysfunction.

5. Mitochondrial dysfunction; nothing new here. We know that mitochondria get abused over time. With failing mitochondria, the increase in free radicals leads to more cell damage and an eventual negative spiral.

6. The longer-lived cells eventually experience epigenetic remodeling. Because some drift more than others, any particular tissue can end up with what is referred to as 'epigenetic mosaicism.' Therefore, some stem cells are more or less capable of doing their jobs. As well, this can lead to a loss of replication plasticity such that certain cell types cannot be refurbished. It can also lead to cancer, for example when a stem cell drifts into uncontrolled reproduction.

7. Changing neighborhood; eventually, as the body ages, so does the niche or stem cell nursery. Secondary to reduced circulation, reduced raw materials, or harmful circulating inflammatory factors or cytokines, the niche is unable to support the cells as they had before. In fact it is well established that systemic inflammatory factors can be detrimental to the stem cell population.

• •

"Aging of niche cells and age-dependent alterations in the acellular components of stem cell niches can cause maladaptive changes in stem cell function."[11]

• •

Thus, the aging stem cell population is a huge component to aging in general.

• •

"The decline in functional capacity and genetic integrity of adult tissue stem cells is thought to be a major factor in the decline in tissue maintenance and the increase in cancer formation during aging."[13]

• •

So, is there any good news in any of this? Luckily there is. And most of it, you have already become familiar with.

How to help the stem cell

1. Overall cell health; keeping the cells as healthy as possible is an obvious first step. Providing them with all the nutrients they need is primary, including the micronutrients that people tend to overlook. There is a theory of micronutrient deficiency of aging, whereby the fast turnover cells are limited by the lack of raw materials. As a result, I'm particularly fond of prenatal vitamins for everyone, regardless of sex (male or female, not the actual action) or an actual state of pregnancy. We build so many new cells each day that it seems that we should treat our new cells as well as we treat fetal cells, such that our stem cells aren't nutrient deficient.

2. Telomerase activity can theoretically be increased with adjuvants, such as astragalus (cycloastrogenol). Lifestyle factors can also improve telomerase activity, including physical exercise, diet, micronutrient supplementation, meditation and yoga.[14]

3. Blocking the effects of chronic inflammation is an easy one. Protecting the microenvironment or stem cell niche can only be beneficial.

4. Enhancing mitochondrial function. We have spent a lot of time on this, but it is important.

• •

"Enhanced mitochondrial function has been associated with improved stem cell function and tissue regeneration in mammals."[11]

Of note, studies have confirmed that in addition to caloric restriction, resveratrol and nicotinamide riboside both activate SIRT3 and 7 which are known to help with hematopoietic stem cell maintenance[9]

• •

5. Inhibition of free radicals

6. Improve autophagy; improving the recycling system begins with cleaning out the old organelles. Studies have shown that a decline in autophagy clearly limits the lifespan of cells.

7. Improving proteostasis; still working on this.

8. Replete the stem cell pool; still working on this as well. There is some evidence that under particular conditions, standard, non-dividing cells can be coaxed back to becoming active stem cells. Scientists don't have a good handle on this yet, but I'm sure they will with time.

I said from the beginning that this was not going to be an exercise/diet book, however, every now and then I have to make exceptions; and this a big one.

It turns out that exercise is great for stem cells. However, so you don't have to take my word for it only, here are the experts:

• •

"Exercise can promote hematopoiesis (regeneration of blood cells) in the aging systemic environment, and increase the proliferative capacity of aged skeletal stem cell, including satellite and mesenchymal stem cells."[15]

"Exercise is associated with increased telomere length."[15]

"Increased running in aged mice has been shown to enhance neural

progenitor proliferation and neurogenesis to a level comparable to that observed in young animals."[15]

"These studies show that a systemic manipulation such as exercise can rejuvenate adult stem cell function across tissues."[15]

• •

As a working example of stem cells in your body, let's look at the skin. In a simplistic model, the integument falls into two main layers; the dermis or thickest layer underneath, and the epidermis, the layer that sits on top.

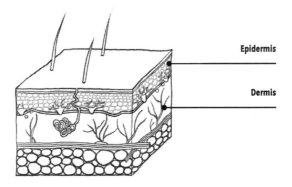

Epidermis

Dermis

Combined, the skin has over 20 types of cells. Most importantly, at least for our discussion, the dermis is replete with mesenchymal stem cells. These produce fibroblasts and adipocytes (fat cells) in addition to a plethora of others. It is the dermal fibroblasts, however, that produce collagen, which is the key structural matrix for the skin.

Meanwhile, stem cells in the epidermal layer produce the stratified epidermis (the dead cells that flake off the top layers of your skin). The melanocytes, cells that produce skin color, originate from additional, specialized melanocyte stem cells.

Thus, there are several different types of stem cells in the skin, and these cells face not only standard stem cell challenges, but they are also especially vulnerable to damage from UVA and B radiation. As a result, these cells carry highly active DNA repair mechanisms, a topic discussed at length in the maintenance chapter.

Therefore, it is no wonder that skin takes a serious beating over time, and can be a very honest reflection of the life someone has led.

As a second example, let's look at the hematopoietic stem cells. These not only make the red blood cells, but the white cells and platelets as well. Within the bone marrow, despite the high turnover of red blood cells, most of the stem cells are in the quiescent state. In fact, of the 11,000 hematopoietic stem cells in the human bone marrow, only about 1,300 are active at any given time.[17] The other thing to note is the loss of differentiation with time; the stem cells are less able to produce B and T cells, which stave off infection.[18] There is also a decline in the B cell repertoire, further increasing the risk of infections. So, with time as the stem cells fail, both infection and blood born cancer risk escalates.

So, in the end, the cell meets its death. Or does it?

Some cells do the right thing and just die. This is called programmed cell death or apoptosis, and occurs when the cell realizes, somehow, that it must go. It just disappears. No fanfare, no nice funeral.

Other cells, however, become the grumpy old men that never leave the factory. They sit around, bitching and moaning and just making life miserable for everyone else. This is called cell senescence.

When a cell becomes senescent, it remains alive, but not helpful. The cells tend to get bigger, with abnormally enlarged, altered mitochondria. As well, these cells secrete bioactive markers that are troublesome. They also secrete degradative enzymes, proteases and inflammatory cytokines as well as other compounds that negatively effect their environment. Referred to as the "Senescence-Associated Secretory Phenotypes," or SASP, the factors are associated with structural tissue damage and organ disfunction.[19]

The immune system is supposed to come to the rescue when this occurs and dispose of the senescent cells, but with age, this fails to occur. This means that, over time, the number of senescent cells increases. This is yet another negative spiral in the world of aging.

Moving along, the goldilocks cells, or those living intermediate periods of time, probably have it the best. They have some of the same challenges as the longest-living cells, but nothing is as severe. It also means, that as a human or organism, these cells and tissues can heal over time.

The shortest-living cells are only challenged by the fact that they are on permanent suicide missions. They generally have a limited, yet key task to perform, and then they perish. Red blood cells for example, are produced in mass quantity. They travel all around the body and take quite a beating. Oxygen and carbon dioxide are constantly jumping on and off, and they have to squeeze through very small spaces.

The real issue with the mass production of red blood cells is the supply chain. For example, hemoglobin, the actual molecule that carries the oxygen requires iron. If the body is deficient in iron, we can't produce enough red blood cells and we are considered anemic. The condition of anemia stresses the rest of the body that requires a constant supply of oxygen.

Thus, there are many different types of cells each facing a variety of challenges. The good news, however, is that we can only improve something when we know what it needs.

And the Kaufmann Protocol knows exactly what that is!

CHAPTER 10:

WASTE MANAGEMENT

For the last factory consideration, we can't overlook the importance of waste management. Like every factory, raw materials and energy are imported, a product is created, and garbage accrues in the process. Generally, this is ignored, but it isn't trivial. You either need to truck it out, bury it or burn it; but you just can't forget about it.

In the human body, waste products come in many forms, some more and some less obvious. Urine and feces are the most obvious of the examples. We drink fluids and consume foods, and the remnants get appropriately excreted.

Less obvious, however is carbon dioxide. We breath in oxygen, and we exhale carbon dioxide. This molecule is actually very acidic. If for some reason you couldn't get rid of it, you would become acidotic and perish.

Even less obvious are the side products of our metabolism. For starters, let's look at glucose and oxygen. Both are interesting substances that we can't live without, but both are also quite detrimental. At some point in time, eons ago when our metabolisms were evolving, both were in short supply and the body did everything it could to catch and retain these vital molecules. The irony, of course now, is that while there is a baseline requirement for both, having a surplus is not beneficial.

Earlier, we talked about oxygen. Without it, people die. Too much however, and the mitochondria and cells suffer from free oxygen radicals and the collateral damage. Too much oxygen can also destroy the stem cell niche.

Glucose is similar. Having evolved in a land where sugars were scarce, the body created very intricate mechanisms to absorb, store and utilize glucose in the body. Perhaps this is why sugar tastes so good to us; the body learned to crave a necessary energy source.

Regardless, when sugars are ingested, they first go to the digestive tract where they are absorbed into the blood stream. The blood travels to the liver where some of it is used immediately, and some is stored for later as fat. When the body is in need, the liver can both send for and utilize this fat. The liver does this by creating new glucose (gluconeogenesis).

When the body consumes too much sugar, fat accumulates. In times of low caloric intake, of course the fat stockpile get reduced. What is even more interesting, however, is that as we age, our genes dictate an increase in the fat storage regardless of the glucose balance. It even changes the location of fat storage. Aging fat, in fact, gets stored near the viscera, or inner organs, and we see this as that middle belly fat (the abdominal tire syndrome) that just will not go away; but alas, this is fixable.

Remember the story of AMP Kinase...

The other necessary part of the glucose story is insulin. Insulin is a protein produced in the pancreas, specifically in the beta-islet cells, that is necessary for getting glucose into cells. Think of this as a doorman for the sugar. Without insulin, it doesn't matter how much sugar you ingest or have in your circulation. It just can't get inside a cell on its own. Under normal circumstances, the pancreas hums along efficiently, creating insulin as the need arises and both molecules act together providing the energy necessary for each and every cell.

There are two basic problems (more than two in reality, but for our purposes, we'll stick to the two) that can arise with this system, referred to as Type I and Type II Diabetes. Type I, aka juvenile, diabetes is an autoimmune disease whereby the body creates antibodies during childhood (usually) which decimate the pancreas and prevent the production of insulin. With little or no insulin available, the glucose levels in the blood rise and rise, but the cells themselves starve. Clearly, this is a serious problem, but, it is one that we are not going to deal with in this book.

Type II diabetes is our big problem and it is multifactorial. People (adults and kids) consume too much sugar (in this country anyway) forcing the body to produce more and more insulin. Thus, increasing amounts of sugar gets stored as fat, and this leads to obesity. In addition, the pancreas gets stressed, as the need continues to escalate, and eventually the production maxes out. The pancreas simply cannot produce enough. With limited insulin, the glucose floats around the vasculature with nowhere to go.

At very high levels in the blood, eventually the sugar acts as a diuretic and the body just starts making more and more urine.

• •

Of note, this was how diabetes was originally diagnosed, the production of sweet smelling urine.

• •

Over time, this excess glucose causes the failure and collapse of almost every body system. Cataracts form in the eyes, nerves die, kidneys fail, tissues can't heal, blood vessels are destroyed; essentially diabetes is a terrible disease.

So, who exactly is diabetic? Over the years, physicians have determined absolute laboratory values of blood sugar to determine who was and who was not diabetic. At some point, they created a category called "pre-diabetic," people who were likely to fall over the edge and into the disease category. Regardless, once labeled with the disease, medications are generally initiated to lower blood sugar. Patients as well, are counseled about diet and exercise.

The threshold of being diabetic or pre-diabetic, however is just an imaginary line. One could argue that almost everyone is pre-diabetic. Interestingly, as we age, almost every sign, symptom and body failure that accompanies diabetes occurs with time. 'Non-diabetic' people may fall below a certain level of blood glucose, but over the course of six, seven or eight decades, even mild glucose levels eventually cause problems.

The question then becomes, why does this happen?

So, it turns out that extraneous glucose, even small amounts, floating around in the blood stream, gets into a lot of trouble. Much like teenagers with nothing to do, they wander from place to place, attach themselves to tissues and assorted structures where they are not needed, and precipitate a slow, yet very destructive condition.

This occurs, as we actually all know, because glucose is sticky. It is sticky in lollypop form, and it is sticky in molecular form. Glucose sticks to pretty much everything it comes into contact with in the body: proteins, lipids, DNA, collagen…almost everything. This process is referred to as non-enzymatic glycation and it is generally considered irreversible, simply meaning that the fusion of glucose to another molecule does not require any help. Once stuck, it does not come off.

A second condition necessary for glycation is oxidative stress, and we have already noted that we humans have a plethora of oxidative stress. In this case, the free radicals, both oxygen and carbonyl species that we addressed previously, accelerate the sticky sugar problem. To make matters worse, the bonding of sugar to these other molecules actually then creates even more free radicals in the process, thus perpetuating the vicious, evil cycle.

In reality, this bonding of sugar to a substrate is a multiple step process whereby the first few steps are reversible, but the last ones are not.

Fair warning, this next section is very science heavy.

Anyway, Louise Camille Maillard first described the glycation reaction in 1912 as a process whereby the carbonyl group on a sugar binds to the free amino residues or amino terminal group of a protein, lipid or a DNA macromolecule. This therefore, is also referred to as the Maillard reaction. By structural, irreversible molecular rearrangement, a more stable keto-amine is formed that is called an Amadori product. This product further morphs through oxidation, dehydration and degradation to yield very stable, but harmful molecules.

• •

Specifically, glycation is the "result of covalent bonding of a free amino group of biological macromolecules with a reducing sugar, which result in the formation of a schiff base that undergoes rearrangement, dehydration, and cyclization to form a more stable Amadori product."[1]

• •

This combination of sugar, usually glucose or fructose, latching onto a molecule under oxidative stressful conditions creates something called an Advanced Glycation End Product or an AGE for short. The more AGEs you have, the more aged you have become.

It should be obvious why this is one of my favorite acronyms. ▶

Because the sugars can bond to almost anything, the label of AGE is very non-specific and can represent a hugely heterogenous pile of molecules. At the present time, there are roughly twenty some different molecules that have been identified as AGEs.

• •

These are divided into 3 main groups: (This isn't really necessary to know, but why not?) Fluorescent cross-linking AGEs, Non-fluorescent cross-linking AGEs, and non-cross linking, non-florescent AGEs. The best known are carboxymethyllysine, pyridine (both non-cross linking) and pentosidine (fluorescent, cross-linking).[2]

• •

Under normal physiologic conditions, the formation of these AGEs can take weeks to months, and tends to affect longer-lived substrates. Collagen, for example is a prime target. The attachment of AGEs to collagen compromises its structural integrity. This phenomena is thus hugely detrimental to whatever structure that particular collagen is supporting (this will be explained more in a bit). Long lasting tissues that get clearly afflicted include nerves, bones, and the lenses in the eyes.

On the other hand, under pathological conditions such as high glucose availability, increased temperature and increased oxidative stress, the reactions can occur over hours and also affect short-lived molecules like hormones and enzymes.[3]

As we have seen, the standard products we have been talking about are called AGEs, when sugars are complexed to proteins. The name cleverly changes when the substrates change. When the sugar attaches to lipids, it is referred to as an Advanced Lipid oxidation End product or ALEs, (another great abbreviation). Attachment to DNA molecules, however has a less clever name simply called DNA-AGEs. The most important thing to realize however, is that whatever the glucose elects to fuse with, the activity of that substance is essentially lost.

Glycation of proteins is considered the biggest problem. As we discussed in a different chapter, proteins are crucial for existence, and thus the unnecessary loss of proteins is a big metabolic drain. With this bonding process, you see structural alterations that effect every aspect of cell life. They are critical for bioenergetics, cellular repair and life in general; and whereas it is very difficult to measure AGEs within our bodies (it is possible, just very expensive), there is one measure that is quite simple to do.

• •

Of note, for those geeks, glucose has a propensity for particular amino acids within the protein; lysine is particularly magnetic.

• •

Because all of the proteins in the plasma get coated with AGEs, from serum albumin to the immunoglobulins, we can choose one and measure it. Luckily, one of these is a very common lab test done for diabetics; HgA1C, or hemoglobin A 1C, a complex with a sugar attached to a hemoglobin molecule. Usually, this measurement allows diabetics to track their glucose control over the course of several months. For non-diabetics, however, the blood test can simply be used as a marker of AGE deposition.

Of note, everyone has a certain degree of glycated hemoglobin. Every animal that utilizes glucose or a sugar as substrate (and has hemoglobin) has some level of glycated hemoglobin. The idea, however, is to get it as low as possible without inflicting any hypoglycemic damage on the body.

• •

The presence of this molecule was identified in 1955 by Kungel and Wallenius, but the idea that protein glycation might be related to aging, and age-related pathologies, wasn't presented until the early 1980s.[4]

• •

All right, so let's be more specific. Some of the important proteins that contribute to our structural integrity include collagen and elastin, among others. These are found in skin, bone and especially in blood vessels. In the walls of our arteries, collagen and elastin provide the strength and flexibility to contain our fluctuating blood pressure, stretching and recoiling as the heart beats.

• •

> *Collagen provides the structural framework, while elastin provides the extensibility. Collagen can stretch about 10%, while elastin can stretch about 200%.*[5]

• •

Over time, i.e., with aging, the structural system fails. Arterial stiffening is a well-described, progressive process that occurs throughout the body, causing high blood pressure and decreased blood delivery to the necessary organs. Whereas this process happens to everyone eventually, it is especially accelerated in diseases such as diabetes.

This occurs, in part, because of our new enemy, the AGEs. Not only do AGEs bind to and prevent individual molecules from acting appropriately, they bond to our structural components and destroy them.

I like to use the example of a piece of fabric with interwoven fibers. The fabric has the ability to stretch a bit in various directions as the fibers slide across each other. If however, you put a drop of superglue on the fabric, the fibers can no longer slide. Instead, they just break. This is exactly what happens to your collagen with age. AGEs stick to the collagen and as a result, the fibers break and the supportive matrix becomes disorganized.

Consequently, the supportive matrix of all of our organs become less than supportive when covered in AGEs. Thus, over time and with increasing accumulations of AGEs, every tissue that is comprised of collagen eventually fails. For example, arteries become progressively stiffer, causing the blood pressure to rise higher and higher. Collagen in the heart gets stiffer as well, and eventually leads to heart failure.

This mechanical demise occurs in many structures throughout our body, and one less deadly but more obvious example is the skin. Over time, our once elastic and beautiful skin loses its ability to retain shape. There is even a test of how well you are aging; the 'pinch test' examines the time it takes for the skin on the back of your hand to retract after it has been tented up by pinching. This is, in essence, a test of the failing support system. Try it, it is really depressing. You simply pinch the skin on the back of your hand and hold it for 5 seconds. The time it takes to return to normal is supposed to predict your functional age.

In fact, this is just more evidence that AGEs really are detrimental.

Anyway, once glycated, the functionality of ALL proteins drop. Enzymes slow down, our faces droop, muscles don't function as well... essentially nothing functions as it should.

DNA, meanwhile, is another favorite target of glycating sugars. This can lead to many forms of DNA damage including single and double-stranded breaks, and mutations such as insertions, deletions, and even transpositions. This happens as the effected DNA gets partially unwound, allowing the double-helix structure to become fragmented.

Science geeks might be interested to note that of the four base pairs found in DNA, the guanosine exhibits the highest rate of glycation. The good news is that we have already learned about DNA repair mechanisms. The bad news however, is that sugar and consequently DNA-AGEs lead to the loss of genomic integrity. This happens quickly in diabetics, but it occurs in all of us with time.

Not only do these harmful molecules float around attacking innocent structures, scientists have even identified cellular receptors that they bind to, and as a result, inflict more cellular damage. Located in tissues as varied as the heart, lung and skeletal muscle, these receptors are also found on individual cells such as macrophages, adipocytes, and even endothelial cells in blood vessel walls.[2] At the moment, there are 3 identified receptors, AGE-R1, AGE-R2, and RAGE, but with time there will probably be more.

One of two things can happen when the AGE complexes to the cells receptor. The first is actually beneficial. The AGE gets incorporated or engulfed by the cell, and then systematically destroyed. Unfortunately, most of the time the second alternative occurs. The AGE lands on the receptor, and triggers undesirable, destructive processes. Specifically, it ignites the inflammatory cascade by activating Nuclear factor- $\kappa\beta$ (a potent inflammatory agent that we've visited before). This then initiates a feedback loop whereby increased NF leads to an increase in the RAGEs, thus leading to even higher levels of inflammation.

As a specific example, RAGE activation of endothelial cells (the inner lining of the blood vessels) triggers an increased permeability of the blood vessel wall. This leakiness allows fluid to escape into the tissues, causing edema. It also allows the entry of lipids into the wall, which is considered the first step in atherosclerosis. This eventually leads to peripheral vascular disease, or a decrease in the blood flow to your necessary parts. RAGE activation also triggers the expression of adhesion molecules, which furthers the progression of the atherosclerosis.

RAGE activation on platelets and white blood cells also stimulate increased production of most inflammatory factors, including (but probably not limited to) IL-1, TNF-α, platelet derived growth factor, and Insulin like Growth Factor.

Ultimately, as we have become aware, this chronic inflammatory state leads to long term harm. Many scientists are in fact convinced that AGEs and the associated RAGEs are the key to understanding atherosclerosis and almost all of diseases associated with the narrowing of blood vessels; strokes, heart attacks, etc.

• •

> *"AGEs interact with Receptor for AGEs (RAGE) leading to oxidative stress and activation of pro-inflammatory pathways, which is believed to be the major cause of glycation associated diseases such as diabetic complications, aging, obesity, inflammation, polycystic ovarian syndrome, ischemic cardiovascular disease, neurodegenerative disorders and cancer."*[6]

• •

Unfortunately, in addition to our internally created AGEs, it turns out we consume or ingest premade AGEs as well. We can inhale their precursors from cigarette smoke, and they are also present in specific foods. Of the total ingested AGEs, it is estimated that we absorb roughly 10 - 30% in our GI tract, and of these, 2/3 are deposited into tissues.

I said from the onset (and repeated frequently) that this was not a book about diet or exercise, but every now and then, I don't seem to have a choice. There are foods or more importantly, methods for preparing foods, that carry increased loads of AGEs.

These include:

1. Highly heated, processed foods
2. Any food that is cooked by browning (mimicking the Maillard reaction)
3. High lipid and protein containing foods
4. Dry heat cooking techniques: fermenting, grilling, frying, roasting, baking, and barbecue

Therefore, real experts suggest that in order to reduce AGE intake, cooking should be restricted to lower temperatures, longer time periods, and using more water while cooking. They particularly recommend boiling, poaching, or steaming.

It turns out that if you restrict the diet of diabetics as to avoid foods and cooking methods that have high levels of AGEs, you can seriously control some of the complications of the diabetes.

While we are discussing food, the type of sugar being consumed is important as well. Interestingly, as much as I've talked about it, glucose is actually a fairly stable sugar with low reactivity. By comparison, fructose is 7.5 times more reactive than glucose in terms of creating AGEs, and perhaps why foods with high fructose as an ingredient tend to be worse for us.[4]

The body, of course has developed ways of eradicating some of these AGEs. For one, we are able to pee them out, but individuals with kidney issues, obviously, cannot. Hemodialysis and peritoneal dialysis can get rid of some AGEs, but that is a topic for another day.

We are also able to break down AGEs in what is called 'extracellular proteolysis,' meaning that outside of the cells, enzymes are roaming around that can reverse the process if caught early. As well, there are receptors for

AGEs on specific cells that cause the AGE to be taken inside the cell and degraded into smaller pieces. The remnants, called second generation AGEs, which are low molecular weight soluble peptides, are then transported to the kidneys and excreted.

As you have probably deduced, the body is unable to dispose of all the AGEs in a timely and efficient manner. This inevitably results in a gradual, but unrelenting accumulation of AGEs. Therefore, as we have seen before, normal aging is just a slower version of what occurs with disease states. These products accumulate faster in diabetics and renal failure patients; but we will reach the same end, under normal conditions, given enough time.

So, we have established that AGEs, ALEs and DNA-AGEs are essentially terrible. The question then of course, is what do we do about them?

1. Prevent the formation of molecules in the first place. Limit sugars and oxidation. All of the substances that reduce the formation and presence of free radicals can help reduce the formation of AGEs. Decreasing sugar intake or lowering blood glucose levels as well, is a no brainer. In fact, a high glucose level not only is a problem unto itself, but it generates even more reactive oxygen species.

2. Accelerate the catabolism or breakdown of these substances.

3. Possibly block the effect of the substances once they are already formed?

Prevention of AGEs

Several steps are involved in the process, making it possible to block the formation somewhere along the pathway.

1. **Aminoguanine:** In 1986, this was the first agent proposed to help in the eradication of AGEs. Whereas the molecular mechanism was and is effective, the side effect profile isn't good. Possible complications include myocardial infarction (heart attack), congestive heart failure, atrial fibrillation (more bad heart stuff), anemia, vasculitis, abnormal liver function and as always, GI upset.

2. **Pyridoxamine:** Considered an AGE formation inhibitor, this agent is a subtype of vitamin B6 and blocks several steps in the formation process.

Spoiler Alert: There's an entire chapter devoted to this in Part 2

• •

"A naturally occurring derivative of B6, (pyridoxamine) has proven to be an effective inhibitor for protein glycation and lipid oxidation both in vitro and in vivo."[8]

• •

3. **Hydralazine:** This medication, used to treat high blood pressure, can actually prevent AGE formation. Remarkably, it can also deglycate or transglycate. This means that the sugar can actually be removed from the afflicted molecule, at least in diabetic mice where it was recently discovered (meaning the sugar from the Schiff base or Amadori product is transferred to something else). This was a phenomenal discovery, but unfortunately hydralazine requires a prescription, and will lower your blood pressure.

• •

"Such compounds (hydrazine and dihydrohydralazine) have attracted considerable interest for their excellent scavenging activity toward reactive carbonyls, and indeed, they have been proven to be therapeutically efficient in preventing AGE and ALE formation in several oxidative-stress based disorders including diabetes, atherosclerosis, and Alzheimers disease."[8]

• •

I am extremely excited by the following experiment, and thus I think that it deserves some special attention.

Diabetic mice were given either aminoguanine or hydralazine while non-diabetic mice served as controls. After fifteen days of treatment, the HgA1C in the hydralazine group was almost reduced to that of the control group. Thus, the once glycated hemoglobin was no longer coated in the sugar complex. Where did the AGEs go? The researchers examined the urine and found hydralazine glucose conjugates. This means that the glucose was removed from the plasma proteins by the hydralazine, and the body was then able to pee them out. Therefore, at least in mice, there is finally evidence that a medication can reverse the glycation process.

• •

"Findings suggest that transglycation can be used as an intervention strategy for the treatment of glycation associated diseases such as diabetes, atherosclerosis, and aging."[6]

• •

4. Alagebrium/ALT-711: This was an agent that was the first (and last for that matter) to be produced and clinically tested for the clinical purpose of breaking down AGEs. The drug made it through promising clinical trials until the company, Alteon, ran out of money. The company was bought in 2007 by Synvista, but they terminated the trials in 2009. So, unfortunately, this type of therapy is presently unavailable.

Other great agents that can positively affect the AGE problem include two of my favorites, metformin and carnosine.

• •

"Peptide derivatives like N-acetyl carnosine with transglycation activity is being used in the eye drop formulation for the treatment of diabetic induced cataract."[6]

• •

These compounds are so remarkable that they have their own chapters later on in the book.

Lipofuscin

In our continuing discussion of waste management, we are going to examine the effects of age on long-lived cells. We alluded to this in earlier chapters, but I will delve into this a little more deeply. Why long-lived cells? Because they don't get replaced, and thus are faced with both the challenge of needing to recycle and the innevitable accumulation of garbage.

As we now know, over time, parts of every older cell get worn out and damaged by life processes. We know that free radicals, oxidants and other toxins cause significant damage. So, eventually, all of the organelles, especially the mitochondria, fail with time. Luckily, as we have seen, various protein and DNA repair mechanisms are in place to repair the damage. In addition to this, the process of autophagy becomes critical.

We touched briefly on autophagy elsewhere, but it deserves a little more attention.

In essence, in order to be recycled, failing cellular structures are engulfed by special vesicles, called lysosomes, which are enzyme-filled sacs within the cell. The interior of the vesicle is acidic, and it contains up to fifty different enzymes that can dissolve pretty much anything. When the lysosome engulfs a cell part, it breaks the pieces down into reusable molecules. This saves in both energy and raw resources.

The lysosome has many other tasks as well, such as being involved in cell signaling, plasma membrane repair, and energy metabolism, but for now the point is that the lysosome is the cell's recycling center.

Despite the high rate of recycling, the reality is that the cell's lysosome cannot break down all of the things it engulfs. Some molecular complexes are just too tough to tear apart. Thus, a small percentage of the digested cellular material remains behind in the vesicle as garbage. It is material that cannot be reused or recycled, and yet the cell can't get rid of it either. What does the cell do? It does what we as humans do...the cell hides the excess garbage in the back corner of the cell where no one will see it.

> Remember the kitchen drawer analogy?

• •

> *"Inherent insufficiency of these degradative processes results in progressive accumulation within long-lived post mitotic cells of biological "garbage," such as indigestible protein aggregates, defective mitochondria, and lipofuscin, an intralysosomal, polymeric, undegradable material."*[9]

• •

OK, not really, but the excess garbage, made of proteins, lipids and metals gets compacted together making it dense and even more non-digestible.

Then, it does nothing; the garbage just sits there, doing nothing, really, just taking up space.

This gunk, called lipofuscin, in fact does several things... by doing nothing.

Number one, it is used as a marker for age. This is not unreasonable. The 'liver spots' that accumulate in the skin as we age are lipofuscin. You see them in almost everyone. You can in fact, laser these spots off if you really want to... I have; and now that you know this, feel free to try it. Unfortunately, lipofuscin doesn't just appear in our skin. It's in some very important tissues; especially your heart, nerves and your brain.

Spots that can't, or really shouldn't be lasered! ▶

• •

Lipofuscin: "An intracellular indigestible material mainly composed of oxidized proteins (30-58%) and lipids (19-51%). It is highly resistant to proteolytic degradation and accumulates in post mitotic cells. The intracellular rate of lipofuscin formation is negatively correlated with the remaining lifespan of cells and increases with age."[10]

"Lipofuscin is a morphological structural entity and is mainly accumulated in post-mitotic cells of the brain. The accumulation of lipofuscin in cells occurs because it is undegradeable and cannot be removed from cells via exocytosis."[11]

• •

Interestingly, we are not the only victims of lipofuscin stashing. It turns out that we have this is in common with innumerable other creatures. In fact, scientists age lobsters by the collection of nervous system lipofuscin. More precise than size or weight, the concentration of this gunk has been shown to be key to aging accuracy in the American Lobster, the European Lobster, the Australian Rock Lobster and even shrimp and crayfish.[12]

Number two, as the cell and lysosomes become overwhelmed with lipofuscin, the cell becomes unable to perform its tasks. Aged animal cells have been noted to be filled about 40% with lipofuscin. One centurion human had motor neurons that were 75% stuffed.[13] Therefore, this can be a real space occupying problem. The lysosomes, becoming increasingly filled, lose their ability to function. Subsequently, they lose the capacity for autophagy.

The broken organelles then, unable to be replaced, continue to function but in a suboptimal manner. Old mitochondria, for example, produce less ATP while creating more and more free radicals. Thus, the cell becomes even more damaged. This negative spiral eventually contributes to death of long-lived cells.

There also seems to be a correlation between the magnitude of reactive oxygen species and the accumulation of lipofuscin. This makes a lot of sense. The more damage that is inflicted on the cell structures by ROS and free radicals, the more the organelles, proteins and lipids need to be replaced or repaired. This places a huge burden on the lysosomes, which then contribute to the ever increasing accumulations of lipofuscin.

• •

"Lipofuscin formation appears to depend on the rate of oxidative damage to proteins, the functionality of mitochondrial repair systems, and the functionality and effectiveness of lysosomes."[13]

"Consequently, the turnover of mitochondria progressively declines, resulting in decreased ATP synthesis and enhanced formation of reactive oxygen species, including further mitochondrial damage and additional lipofuscin formation."[9]

• •

This theory correlating oxidative damage, lipofuscin and aging was examined in our classic rat population.[14] Not unexpectedly, they demonstrated that lipid peroxidation and lipofuscin concentrations increased with age, while our friendly antioxidant enzymes, superoxide dismutase and glutathione peroxidase, decreased with age.

It would seem that the collection of lipofuscin is therefore an inevitable part of aging. It happens to lobsters, it happens to us.

• •

" ...the intracellular rate of lipofuscin formation is negatively

correlated with the life expectancy of a post mitotic cell and increases with age: The higher the rate of intracellular lipofuscin accumulation over time, the shorter the future lifetime of the cell."[13]

• •

Amazingly enough, however, there are actually ways to reduce its accumulation, and in some situations, actually get rid of it.

This brings us to another of my absolute favorite substances, curcumin. Again, there will be an entire chapter on this stuff a little later, but I think it's important to mention this particular aspect of the substance while we're on the subject.

There was a great study that fed curcumin to rats for a month. Overall, they demonstrated a significantly decreased level of lipofuscin deposition in four different regions in the brain in both old and young rats. Truly amazing!

In fact, there were a lot of really cool stats in this study, but the best ones are the following: In old rats (24 months old) that had only one month of curcumin, lipofuscin decreased 60% in the cerebellum, 40% in the medulla, 24% in the cerebral cortex and 18% in the hippocampus. So, the curcumin didn't just decrease the accumulation of the lipofuscin, it actually removed some of it.

Don't just skim over these numbers; think about them for a minute. These decreases are truly impressive. We have no idea if this extrapolates to humans as we don't have too many volunteers willing to have their brains dissected, but even if it only helped a fraction of what it did in rats, we still win. Any improvement can only help us.

What tissues are we specifically referring to here? Clearly, the brain is important, but we are also talking about other neurons, cardiac muscle, skeletal muscle, pancreatic cells and retinal pigment cells.[15]

Thus, all of these long-lived tissues and organs are considered high risk for failure over time. Deterioration of cardiac muscle leads to heart disease, pancreatic deficiency leads to diabetes, and the breakdown of retinal cells leads to vision loss. Obviously, there are other reasons for these organs to fail, but if we can decrease at least a fraction of the negative insults, we gain just a little more ground.

PART 2

Welcome to the second half of the book. If you've gotten this far, you now have a reasonably good idea of why you and your cells are aging.

So, now for the good part. What can we do to fix these issues?

To answer this question, I have reviewed and trialled innumerable substances in the hope of achieving the best and most credible list; and by trialled, I mean, by Me. I have personally tried each and every one of these substances…and a zillion more on top of this. My close friends are waiting for me to die of some crazy disease or toxicity, but so far I am healthier and better off than I have ever been.

The other thing you will realize is that I seem to use a few words interchangeably, but, I really am not. A supplement, for example can only be a supplement if you already have some in your body. You are supplementing your endogenous quantities. An adjuvant, meanwhile, is something you don't already have. It is a brand new, traceable substance. Therefore, you will find a collection of both of these types of substances.

As is standard, some people will agree with my list, some people will not. Some folks will even be disappointed that their favorite supplement didn't make it. (Don't get too upset, there will be more agents on the website and the App.)

You will have heard of some of these, others may be brand new.

As always, however, there are a few things you need to consider as you dive into this list.

1.   I have no preference toward natural substances versus unnatural ones. If they are efficacious, fabulous! They are all described in detail, so if you have a predilection one way or another, at least you can make your own, educated decisions.

2.   This is a book about aging and aging only. This is not a book about everything that might be good for you. There are a zillion substances that will help you with a variety of problems. There are many substances, for example, that may make you think better, but those didn't qualify. Neither did those that only increased muscle mass or exercise endurance. If these qualities are a side effect, however, of those that are included…then bonus! The list had to be exclusive and there had to be a cut off.

3. Before implementing any of these substances, I strongly recommend that you check with your personal physician first. Some of these substances can negatively interfere with prescription medications. Just know that your physician might think that you are a bit crazy. Feel free to give him/her a copy of the book!

4. There may be other substances out there that are protective against aging. I used real, scientific journals as the only source of information. Just because you read something on Wikipedia or saw it on Dr. Oz...it doesn't count. It is also possible that new and phenomenal substances are on the horizon. By the time you read this, I could have just missed the next superstar.

So, alas, I have chosen 15 substances that I believe will stave off aging. Why 15? Because they all stood out for a particular reason. I felt terrible throwing a few out, but they just weren't good enough.

Because this subject is a bit complex and overwhelming, I have created a systematic process for taking on this challenge. First, I have rated these agents in each of the seven categories of aging that you just read about. Thus, at the end of each of the following chapters, you will see a "Kaufmann Rating". The scale is from 0 to 3 in each of the seven tenets of aging. Zero means the substance has no effect in a certain category. A rating of three means the agent has a strong effect, and the research is extremely convincing. A score of 1 to 2 falls somewhere in between. Therefore, each substance ends up with a seven digit rating number, called the Kaufmann Rating.

As an example, the Kaufmann Rating for Astaxanthin is **0.3.0.0.2.0.0.**

This is interpreted as meaning the following:

There is no effect at all in the Information system/Genetic category, thus the first zero.

Mitochondria, the second category, rates a 3.

There are no effects in the categories of Pathways or Quality control.

In the Security or Immune system, astaxanthin rates a 2.

Lastly, there are no effects on individual cells or in waste management.

Following this idea, it becomes obvious that several agents must be utilized in order to cover all of the aging challenges. Thus, the easiest way to keep track is to follow the table that's in the back of the book. If you sum all of the points in a certain category, you will know how effectively you are combating age. If you have missed a category or two, you will need to rethink your strategy.

But, alas, it has happened again. I'm getting ahead of myself.

The next section reviews the agents, and then finally at the end, we talk strategy.

CHAPTER 11:

THE ENIGMA OF RESVERATROL AND ITS LESSER KNOWN COUSIN, PTEROSTILBENE

Resveratrol is quite impressive, yet also quite confusing. It seems to be omnipotent at times, and useless otherwise. The substance is very old, yet very young. It makes things that are bad for you seemingly good for you; and even if you consume just a little, big things seem to happen. The word paradox is frequently used with resveratrol, but I think that enigma is apt.

The Riddler would have a field day with this agent!

Resveratrol, a component of Japanese knotweed, has been used medicinally for just over 2,000 years. It has been sited in Ayurvedic, Japanese and traditional Chinese medicine as a treatment for fungal infections, cardiovascular disease, gastrointestinal disorders, diabetes and general inflammation. Even today, Itadori tea, a rich source of resveratrol, is made out of knotweed, and used as an herbal remedy for heart disease and stroke.

Once endemic to East Asia, Japan, China and Korea, Japanese knotweed has now migrated into the United States; but rather than appreciate the plant for its health benefits, it has been categorized as one of the worst invasive plant species ever.[1]

Clearly, we have failed to appreciate what is growing in our own backyards!

The substance was first isolated in 1939 from the roots of the white hellebore plant that is also found in the East. Of note, parts of the plant are known to contain highly toxic steroidal alkaloids, and thus it is classified as poisonous. The roots on the other hand, are considered medicinal and used for treating malaria, jaundice, diarrhea and headaches.

This substance was little known to the western world until the 1990s, when scientists starting referring to something called the 'French Paradox.' The French, as is well known, consume a plethora of fatty foods, especially cheese, and smoke cigarettes. They also drink a lot of red wine. They should, by all estimates, be overweight drunks with cardiovascular disease. But, alas, they are not.

Extensive investigations ensued, eventually reaching the conclusion that the substance responsible was resveratrol, found in abundance in red wine. It is also present in blueberries, blackberries, mulberries, peanuts and over seventy different types of plants. Being present in wine makes the substance a bit sexy, and thus more popular.

I'm not above promoting the medicinal benefits of a good buzz

Of note, the skin of the grape contains the greatest content of the active compound. Therefore, there is far more resveratrol in red than white wine as the grape skins are not utilized in the production of whites. So, alcohol, that in general is not a friend to your health, can in fact be beneficial in this circumstance.

So what is this stuff, really?

3,5,4'-trihydroxy-trans-stilbene

I know, a really dull scientific name; but, importantly, it is a stilbene.

As well, it is a polyphenol and a phytoalexin, aka a substance produced by plants when said plant gets stressed out. When particular plants are exposed to environmental challenges such as fungal infections, UV radiation, or exposure to a toxic metal for example, the plant produces the substance as a way to protect itself.

Resveratrol, as well, is fat soluble or lipophilic. This means that it can enter cell membranes which are composed of lipids. In fact, resveratrol generally localizes in the outer leaflet of the lipid bilayer.[2]

Unfortunately, the bioavailability is low. This means that resveratrol gets metabolized rather quickly after being absorbed, and thus lasts in your body for an extremely limited period of time. Even so, as we will see, resveratrol seems to do many beneficial things in the short time it has available.

Back to chemistry...

Resveratrol is composed of 2 phenol rings connected by 2 carbons. The arrangement of the carbons can be either in a cis or trans conformation, which doesn't make that much difference except that the trans seems to be more active. This is only important in that you will notice the trans notation clearly advertised on the label if you elect to purchase the adjuvant.

Anyway, resveratrol was explored in a backwards fashion. People were obviously consuming it in vast quantities, thus ruling out the need for safety tests; and clearly, it was beneficial, but why?

It turns out that resveratrol is a powerhouse among our anti-aging adjuvants. Like many of the others we will discuss, it has a panoply of actions. In fact, because it is so busy, it has been described as a 'Promiscuous Molecule.'[3]

No wonder the French like it so much!

DNA/Information systems: Telomere enhancer

There is evidence that resveratrol can positively effect telomere length.[2] It was found to promote the expression of 'telomere-maintenance factors' such as the helicase gene. It was also discovered to activate human telomerase activity in pulmonary microvascular endothelium cells as well as aortic smooth muscle cells.[4]

How significant this property turns out to be is unknown at the moment; but longer telomeres are always a good thing!

Mitochondria/Energy systems: Direct and Indirect free radical scavenger and antioxidant

While not its strongest attribute, resveratrol does act as a free radical scavenger. More importantly, however, resveratrol indirectly reduces the radicals and oxidants by triggering an increase in the activity of catalase, superoxide dismutase, gluathione peroxidase, and glutathione S-transferase. This is essential as we know that the bodies innate antioxidants drop dramatically with age.

Pathways: SIRTUIN activator

This is the category where resveratrol really shines. Activation of the sirtuin family is crucial to anti-aging, and resveratrol is one of the few truly efficacious agents that we have. In fact, resveratrol turns on the SIRTs in two separate ways. One, it can directly act on the SIRT gene to initiate the sirtuin family cascade. Secondly, it activates AMP Kinase, which subsequently acts on the sirtuin family. Either way, there is definitive proof that resveratrol activates the sirtuins, even increasing their activity up to ten fold.[5]

• •

> *Resveratrol belongs to a prestigious group of substances called STACs or sirtuin activating compounds.*

• •

This quality is exceptionally beneficial because in case you don't recall, "sirtuin activity is linked to gene repression, metabolic control, apoptosis and cell survival, DNA repair, development, inflammation, neuroprotection, and healthy aging."[6]

Of the seven mammalian SIRTs, the question is then: Which ones? So far, we only know about SIRT1, 3 and 4. However, research in this area is young, so don't cite this statement in a few years, as it's bound to change.

Quality Control: Indirect activator of DNA repair mechanisms

This was mentioned briefly in the above section, but it is important enough to mention again. Acting through the sirtuin pathways, the DNA repair process is augmented.

• •

> *"It was shown that resveratrol can modulate the activity of SIRT1, a critical deacetylase that impacts the acetylation status of p53, forkhead proteins, and DNA repair enzymes."*[1]

• •

Immune system/Security: Anti-inflammatory

One of our tenants of aging is the upregulation of the inflammatory component that is considered responsible for innumerable disease states. These include, as we have discussed before, infection, injury, atherosclerosis, diabetes mellitus, obesity, cancer, osteoarthritis, age-related macular degeneration, demyelination, and neurodegenerative diseases.[7]

Specifically, resveratrol in known to reduce C-reactive protein, Tumor Necrosis Factor, and cyclooxygenase-1 and 2 in both cell cultures and real people.

• •

> *Other COX-2 inhibitors include EGCG, Curcumin, Aspirin, Diclofenac, and Ibuprofen.*

> *Scientists examined endometrial cells from women suffering from painful endometriomas, which is actually a very common problem. These cells were found to be remarkably responsive to treatment with resveratrol. Inflammatory markers such as TNF-α and IL-8*

were suppressed, while SIRT1 was upregulated.[8] Anyway, it would be fabulous if drinking red wine actually helped with endometriosis.

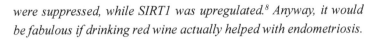

Individual Cell Health: Stem cell activator

There is great evidence in this category. It turns out that resveratrol activates mesenchymal stem cells to produce better bone; more about this is addressed in the bone section below. As a teaser:

"Acting at the level of human mesenchymal stem cells, resveratrol promotes spontaneous osteogenesis or bone formation."[9]

There is also tremendous evidence that resveratrol positively effects multiple types of dental stem cells as well.

Waste Management: Glucose reduction

Blood glucose reduction by resveratrol is very well documented. In human clinical trials, resveratrol significantly improved glycemic control, reduced HgA1C levels and insulin levels.

Why is this waste management? As you might recall, less glucose in the body leads to fewer AGE products. This means less cellular garbage that needs to be cleaned up.

Now that we know that resveratrol works in innumerable mysterious ways, let's look at which organs are most benefited.

"Its effects range from the neuroprotective to the nephroprotective, including cardiovascular, neuronal, and antineoplastic responses as

a part of its broad spectrum of action."[5]

Resveratrol actions "include the prevention of cardiovascular diseases, anti-cancer potential, neuroprotective effects, homeostasis maintenance, aging delay, and a decrease in inflammation."[10]

• •

Cardiovascular

The reality, of course, is that the cardiovascular benefits of resveratrol is what peaked everyone's interest in the first place. We have learned, however, that these benefits are wide ranging, and that heart function, blood pressure and the risk for atherosclerosis are all improved. Specifically, resveratrol limits platelet adhesion, promotes coronary artery vasorelaxation, and even reduces the incidence of heart arrthymias.[10]

Molecular targets for such improvement are thought to include AMP Kinase, COX-1, thromboxane A2, ICAM, NF-$\kappa\beta$ and SIRT1.

Over the years, there have been myriad human studies concerning the cardiovascular system, and there have been many different outcomes. Using a wide range of doses over a wide range of times and examining different variables, the outcomes of studies have been hard to interpret. Some studies showed absolute benefits, while others did not. The paradox continues, but let's leave this category on a positive note:

• •

"Resveratrol treatment provides far ranging cardiovascular protection by improving both cardiac function and architecture, while decreasing vascular effects such as platelet clumping, ischemia-reperfusion injury, and atherosclerosis."[5]

• •

Bone

It turns out that bone is a prime target for resveratrol, but allow me to illustrate with a few simple quotes:

• •

"In one study, it induced osteogenesis, prevented osteoarthritis, and counteracted age related bone loss."[1]

"Data suggest that resveratrol mediates bone building by stimulation of osteoblastic and inhibition of osteoclastic activities."[1]

Enough said! ▶

• •

Dental

This section means a lot to me, thus a short personal detour. After undertaking my adjuvants and supplements (all of them) for about 6 months, I had a standard dental appointment. Following the regular examination and x-rays, the dentist couldn't help but ask what I had done to myself. Everything in my mouth had apparently improved, especially my gums and the alveolar bone density (the bone in which the teeth are embedded). After another 6 month interlude with the same agents, I

And she wasn't referring to the use of foul language! ▶

showed even further amelioration. She declared I had the mouth of a 20 year old!

I was thrilled, of course, but I really had no idea which adjuvant was responsible. I concluded at that moment that my general cellular health had improved, and so my mouth should follow suit; but further research convinced me that while my premise was probably true, I now believe it was the resveratrol more than anything else (and its cousin pterostilbene, to be discussed shortly) that was responsible.

Let's get back on track…

For whatever reason, scientists set out to examine the effects of resveratrol on dental stem cells. It turns out that there are several types of such stem cells, including periodontal ligament stem cells and apical papilla stem cells (those that make the teeth). In the study, both were found to respond positively to the adjuvant. Resveratrol promoted cell proliferation, which gradually increased over time. As well, markers of healthy tooth development and upkeep, such as mineralization, osteopontin, osteocalcin (and other things no one but dentists need know), were all found to increase over time.[11]

Neurologic

Because resveratrol is lipid soluble, it is able to cross the blood brain barrier. This is a very real barrier that separates the blood flow from the brain tissue as it flows through the cranium. The barrier functions to keep toxins and unwanted molecules out of the brain.

So, we know that resveratrol can get directly into the brain, but why is this important?

The brain is a very special organ that is extremely vulnerable for several reasons. The brain uses more oxygen per unit of tissue than any other and has higher energy requirements. This means the brain is exposed to very high levels of oxidative stress and free radicals. The brain also has a very high lipid content, which means that lipid peroxidation is a very real problem.

In innumerable mammal studies, including humans, resveratrol has been found to be neuroprotective, especially in the hippocampus.

Eighteen-month-old rats (reasonably old, for a rat) were given resveratrol at a dose of 20 mg/kg for sixty days. After decapitation and dissection, the hippocampal area in the brain demonstrated an increase in the dendritic length and spine density of the pyramidal neurons. The details of this are not too important, but suffice it to say that the resveratrol created better nerves.[13]

In a primate model using gray mouse lemurs, and following eighteen months of treatment (200 mg/ kg/day), several measurable neurologic parameters had improved. These included increased spacial memory performance, spontaneous locomotor activity, and working memory.

Turning to people, overweight, older individuals were treated with 200 mg per day for six months. Whereas they weren't open to decapitation, they were subjected to multiple scanning techniques and memory tests. It turns out that their word retention after 30 minutes was significantly improved, and they also showed increases in the hippocampal functional connectivity.[14]

Fat

Resveratrol seems to have no end to its powers. Remarkably, it also helps with fat reduction, which is an unexpected, but extremely cool attribute. It turns out that mice on resveratrol had a 33% reduction in inguinal fat as compared to control mice, despite similar food and water intakes.

In another study, eighteen male mice, fed a high fat diet with resveratrol for 2 months had reduced body fat and reduced total cholesterol compared to controls. Referring back to the inflammatory section, TNF-α, IL-6 and NF-$\kappa\beta$ were also diminished.

As for humans, we have only gotten as far as cell cultures, but, when incubated with resveratrol, human fat or adipose cells see an increase in lipolysis, meaning there is a breakdown of fat and triglycerides. There is also a reduction in lipogenesis or fat formation. Scientists have postulated that the substance may help with mild weight loss, but there is no proof quite yet.[15]

Ovary

Men, feel free to skip this next section. It's interesting, but doesn't really have any personal applications.

Normal ovarian aging and the beginning of menopause involves a remarkable (and depressing) decline in the pool of follicles and oocytes (egg cells) as well as the quality of those oocytes. As eggs get older, the DNA replication process fails. This isn't unexpected as the energy requirement to copy the DNA over and over is extremely high, and puts a huge burden on the ovarian mitochondria. With time and failing mitochondria, the DNA replication process starts to fail. This is thought to be why abnormal chromosomes arise more frequently in mothers of advanced age. The DNA replication system either can't make an exact copy, the checking proteins fail, or the cell can't pull the two copies apart completely when the cell divides into two. Therefore, with aging, the rate of miscarriages rise as well as the rate of children being born with abnormal chromosome patterns.

Resveratrol treated lady mice were found to have a greater number of ovarian follicles, and had better, and more numerous oocytes. As well, the telomerase activity and telomere length in the older, treated mice was similar to that of the younger, untreated mice.

In a study of lady pigs and their oocytes, resveratrol increased the ATP or energy content of the oocytes, and protected them from common aging defects, such as chromosomal anomalies or spindle defects.

Scientists believe these effects are mediated through the action of resveratrol on the sirtuin family. We know, in fact, that SIRT1 and SIRT3 are expressed in the mammalian oocyte, and serve as sensors and coordinators of crucial activities during egg development. We think that they protect against an age-dependent decline in fertility by increasing the ovarian follicular reserve, ovarian lifespan, and preventing oocyte apoptosis.

Resveratrol, therefore, inhibits the aging process in the ovary, i.e., it has a 'fertility staying effect.' It limits follicular atresia, increases the ovarian reserve and prolongs the ovarian lifespan (at least in rats).[16]

Why is this a good thing?

For one, the ovary should be considered a microcosm of aging in general. If we can keep oocytes alive and prospering, maybe the process will work for other systems as well.

Secondly, and whereas menstruation is not the most desirable body function, menopause is not good for us as we age. Postmenopausal women experience significantly higher medical problems then premenopausal women. There-fore, more time before menopause may be beneficial in this regard.

Eyes

The eye is an extension of the brain, and like the brain, sight utilizes high amounts of energy and oxygen. As well, its exposure to radiation is huge. Thus, vision fails with time; we all know this. In the disease world, Age-Related Macular degeneration is an extremely common issue with age, as its name suggests. The retina is attacked by continuously high levels of oxidation, and it has been found, not surprisingly, that it is made worse by smoking. Indeed, tobacco combustion contains an extremely high concentration of free radicals and toxic compounds that significantly contribute to vision loss as the eyes are quite close to the mouth.

Resveratrol, of course, has been found to be protective for this disease as well. Not only did studies show that the adjuvant could reduce the production of free radicals in the tissue, it also increased the intrinsic production of superoxide dismutase, glutathione peroxidase, and catalase. Thus, a decline in vision, or at least Age-Related Macular Degeneration can be postponed or avoided.

Resveratrol was also found to be protective for the lens. Deterioration, of course, causes presbyopia (the inability to see up close with advancing age) at best, and disabling cataracts at worst. Recently, it has been found that resveratrol can benefit these cells as well.

Anti-cancer

As I have said before, I am not an oncologist, and therefore I am hesitant to suggest any form of treatment for cancer. However, resveratrol has been found to be beneficial for colon, skin and breast cancers.

Aging?

• •

"Although scarce, studies addressing the anti-aging effects of resveratrol generally suggest that they are exerted via inhibition of oxidative stress, down regulation of inflammatory levels, enhancement of SIRT1 expression and sirtuin-regulated downstream pathways rather than SIRT1 activity."[17]

Studies on mice have found that resveratrol generally improves their health (right before we decapitate them) "showing a marked reduction in signs of aging, including reduced albuminuria and cataract formation, decreased inflammation, and apoptosis in the vascular endothelium, increased aortic elasticity, greater motor coordination, and preserved bone mineral density."[6]

• •

Problems

Our paradoxic molecule seems simply amazing, as it should, but there are limits to its actions based on its low bioavailability. Meaning simply, the amount that gets into your system is low, and the length of time it remains is minimal.

Studies have shown that somewhere between 15 to 70% of ingested resveratrol is bioavailable and the dose lasts 30 to 180 minutes. Realizing these are huge ranges, this is not uncommon for the substance.

It also turns out that there is a huge variability in bioavailability between different individuals without a clear reason either. As well, morning intake demonstrates a higher bioavailability.[18]

But who drinks wine in the morning?

Of the molecules of resveratrol that are absorbed from the gut, they are immediately delivered to the liver and processed. Most of them get conjugated (linked) to glucuronide or sulfate. Of the remainder, most get bound to lipoproteins, usually LDL, or albumin. Thus, very little resveratrol is actually free and available.

Because of the poor bioavailability, but knowing that resveratrol is tremendously useful and thus profitable, many researchers are trying to molecularly package it to improve its status. Innumerable concoctions of nano- and micro-emulsions are presently being formulated.

Of these, ResVida and Longevinex have in fact demonstrated improved bioavailability. Another micronized version of resveratrol, SRT 501, was at one time produced by GlaxoSmithKline. It was discontinued during phase II trials however, when multiple myeloma patients on the medication developed kidney failure. It was not clear if this issue was related to the drug, but side effects were not tolerated either, including nausea and vomiting. Thus, SRT 501 is only a footnote in history.

Disregarding the negatives of resveratrol, the question remains: How much to take?

Based on the French Paradox of wine intake, approximate resveratrol intake has been estimated. In France, where on average a consumer drinks roughly 43.4 liters of wine per year, of which 31.7 liters per year are red, that would work out to 70 mg of resveratrol per year or 0.2 mg/

day. This in fact, is a tiny amount (average red wine: 1.9 +/-1.7 mg/liter).

On the other end of the spectrum, so called experts recommend 12.5 mg/kg, which for a standard person of 70 kg is 875 mg per day and extrapolation from animal studies recommends about 1 gm per day.

Some studies utilize doses up to 2.5 to 5 gm per day, but these tend to precipitate uncomfortable GI side effects.

The reality? There is no known optimal dose.

Meet the cousin of Resveratrol.... Pterostilbene

Secondary to the poor bioavailability of resveratrol, its once under appreciated cousin, pterostilbene, has recently seen a burst of interest and been thrown into the spotlight.

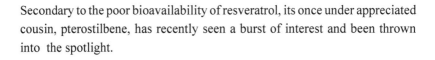

> *"a kind of extra-potent version of resveratrol"[19]...*

The substitution of a hydroxy group with a methoxy group alters the molecule from resveratrol to pterostilbene, and serves to improve the transport into cells as well as increase its metabolic stability. Thus, a slightly different molecule that is not as quickly metabolized.

While the studies on pterostilbene are certainly not as numerous as those on resveratrol, it is believed that the metabolic actions are very similar.

> *"The benefits of pterostilbene are vast and include neuroprotection, inhibition of malignancy, attenuation of atherosclerosis, protection against hemolysis and liver disease, and metabolic regulation of DM and hyperlipidemia."[20]*

This stilbene, however, is not sexy. It is definitely more of the reliable cousin variety. Not too flashy, but certainly around when you need it. While it too is found in many plants including *Pterocarpus marsupium* heartwood, (thus the name) and red sandal wood trees from India, its most prevalent source is blueberries. Blueberries are cute and such, but sex appeal has never been a strong point.

Being a stilbene, pterostilbene is also a phytoalexin and is thus created when the plant is exposed to stress. Again, this could be from a virus, bacteria, fungus, or excessive UV radiation.

The really good news is that pterostilbene has better bioavailability. In a rat study, the numbers were amazing. While resveratrol had a 20% bioavailability (meaning that only 1/5 of what you ingested was actually helpful), pterostilbene demonstrated a high 80%. That is truly significant. Pterostilbene also demonstrated higher blood levels of the free substance as well as some of the lesser active metabolites. Thus, more is simply available.[21]

In a human study, the amount of time the substances were measurable in the blood was compared after an oral dose. In terms of the half life of the molecules, resveratrol was measurable for a measly 14 minutes, while pterostilbene lasted 105.[22]

Thus, pterostilbene is more available, and it lasts a lot longer.

In trying to compare the two substances, I've put together a list that represents the research to date. This changes almost daily, so again, take it for what it is worth.

Pros

Anti-fungal: The cousin was found to be five to ten times more effective than resveratrol against fungus.

Skin: Pterostilbene demonstrated greater skin protection from UV radiation if applied topically.

Cons

Anti-Inflammatory: In some studies, the activity against the COX-1 and 2 cytokines was weaker than resveratrol. It is, however, clearly active against most of the common cytokines including TNF-α, IL-4, IL-1β.

Roughly equivalent

Antioxidant/Free radical scavenging: Pterostilbene increases the expression of superoxide dismutase, catalase, total glutathione, glutathione peroxidase, and glutathione reductase.[20]

Neurologic preservation: Pterostilbene acts to preserve cognitive function and working memory. In a rat study, pterostilbene was effective in reversing cognitive behavioral deficits, and it improved the age-related decline in dopamine release; and because we can decapitate and measure rat brains, this improved working memory was clearly correlated with pterostilbene levels in the hippocampus. Thus, higher levels of pterostilbene were clearly better.[23]

Lipid lowering properties

Anti-diabetic properties

Cancer: These are thought to include gastric, colon, liver, skin, pancreas, lung and breast malignancies.

Cardiovascular Disease

Fat lowering ability

Not definitive

Sirtuin: We know that pterostilbene activates SIRTUINs, but there are no head to head comparisons.

Unlike Violet from Willy Wonka, you will not turn into a giant blueberry ▶ The other good news is that there appear to be no side effects of pterostilbene.

That's one big berry smoothie! ▶ The recommended dose is about 50 to 150 mg BID or two times a day. Average blueberries contain about 9.9 to 15.1 microgram/kg fresh weight of pterostilbene; you therefore would need to consume a lot of blueberries to obtain necessary quantities. Actually, 100 mg is estimated to be about 5,000 cups of blueberries.

Thus, instead of eating millions of blueberries, pterostilbene is of course available in pill form. Most of the available pterostilbene, however, for better or worse, is actually produced in a laboratory and not extracted from plants. Manufacturers claim this makes it more pure, which is actually true. However, if you are looking for a healthy, natural adjuvant, you may have to overlook this small detail.

In fact, Chromodex, which also manufactures nicotinamide ribosome or Niagen, also makes PteroPure, a very popular version of pterostilbene.

The company Elysium, is so impressed with this stuff that they make only one product, called Basis. This is a combination of Niagen and pterostilbene. With six Nobel prize winners on their board, they may be onto something.

Regardless, I'll let the experts sum it up:

• •

> *"Pterostilbene, (more lipophilic and showing higher in vivo bioavailability) appears superior to Resveratrol in practically all comparable studies performed to date."*[24]

> *"Pterostilbene, a methoxylated analog of Resveratrol, is gradually gaining more importance as a therapeutic drug owing to its higher lipophilicity, bioavailability, and biological activity than Resveratrol."*[25]

> *"Pterostilbene is attributed to have anti-diabetic, anti-cancer, anti-inflammatory and antiobesity activity and known to have antioxidant activity comparable to Resveratrol."*[25]

• •

So, which one to take? Resveratrol or Pterostilbene? The choice is yours.

Kaufmann Number: 2.3.3.3.2.2.1

CHAPTER 12:

ASTAXANTHIN

I have
several, as
you will
learn! ▶ Born of humble means, astaxanthin is perhaps one of my favorite substances.

The side product of an almost omnipresent algae, it is created in anger, but imparts a calming effect on biological systems... including us. I think of it as an antidote to anger - soothing, but subtle.

The story begins in the green muck of a birdbath, in ephemeral rain pools, and in fact in most small, temporary freshwater bodies. The unicellular biflagellate green cell, *Haematococcus Pluvialis*, is the main producer of astaxanthin, so we are going to focus on this little being. This one-celled organism lives all over the world; mostly Europe, Africa, North America and parts of India, but always in small bodies of water. It has been found in brackish waters on coasts, in freshwater basins filled with melted snow, dried fountains in Bulgaria and even fishponds in Romania.[1]

This single-celled being is usually green, as you have probably surmised having seen overgrown birdbaths, and it is pretty resilient. What is remarkable, however, is what the algae does when it gets angry. Under unfavorable or stressful conditions, the macrozooids lose their flagella, and get puffed up. Then, they begin producing astaxanthin in small lipid droplets that accumulate in the cytoplasm. Turning the cells bright red, the cell is now able to withstand the extreme environmental conditions that angered it in the first place. Somehow, this miraculous red substance is able to protect the cell.[1]

A few red globules in a single-celled organism doesn't seem like it might do much on the global scale, but amazingly it does. This red substance becomes incorporated into the food chain, and is the basis for almost all of the red we see in crustaceans, fish and birds. It is the red in salmon, lobsters, crabs and shrimp. It is in the feathers of Roseate Spoonbills. It is in the eyes of quail. Most importantly, it gets into us.

Within our bodies, astaxanthin does the same thing it does in the algae from which it came. Cellular stress to an algae can range from a high salinity environment, a nitrogen deficiency, or even high temperatures. Stress to a human cell can be envisioned by many of the things we have already discussed, including oxidative damage and free radicals. Astaxanthin acts by calming down an irritated system, and promoting cellular survival. It quenches free radicals, blocks damage from oxidative stress and it acts as an anti-inflammatory. It can alleviate preexisting trauma, and it can block the onset of new destruction. In terms of aging, it can actually repair some of the cellular damage that has accumulated, and it can help to control cellular survival going forward.

Let's back up a bit, because as usual… I'm getting ahead of myself.

Astaxanthin is a xanthophyll carotenoid, which basically means a plant pigment that is usually very colorful. Other substances in this family include carotenes which are yellow to orange, beta carotenes which are green to yellow, lutein which is yellow, zeaxanthin which makes Indian corn yellow and lycopene that makes tomatoes red. Astaxanthin is red as well, but it is bright red; intensely red. As I mentioned, it is the substance that makes lobsters and crabs red.

The other thing that makes this molecule different is its structure. Formally called 3,3'-dihydroxybeta, beta-carotene-4,4'-dione, or $C_{40}H_{52}O_4$, it is a long molecule consisting of a chain of carbons in the middle with an ionone ring on each end; essentially it resembles a simple chain bracelet with a circular clasp. The conjugated double bonds at the center of the molecule are responsible for the red color, but alas, just a geeky detail.

What makes this molecule so special? The simple fact that it is capable of doing so many amazing, positive things in the body without any real side effects.

Astaxanthin is many things:

Mitochondria / Energy systems: Antioxidant & free radical scavenger

What is the difference you ask? This is a key category for astaxanthin, so I'm going to go into a little bit of detail here.

An antioxidant is a molecule that inhibits the oxidation of other molecules. Oxidation is a chemical reaction that can produce free radicals, leading to chain reactions that may damage cells.

A free radical scavenger, meanwhile, is a molecule that is able to destroy free radicals. The term 'free radical' refers to a molecule that has one or more unpaired electrons. This makes them very unstable, and they move through the bloodstream, taking electrons from other cells or giving away unpaired ones.

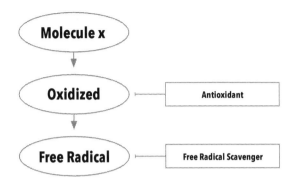

· ·

Astaxanthin "serves as a safeguard against oxidative damage by various mechanisms, like quenching of singlet oxygen; scavenging of radicals to prevent chain reactions; preservation of membrane structure by inhibiting lipid peroxidation; enhancement of immune system function and regulation of gene expression."[2]

· ·

For simplicity sake, we are going to clump the ideas of free radical scavenging and antioxidation together, as the specific sites of action are sometimes difficult to pin down. As the result is the same, it is going to be easier to treat this as a single item.

So anyway, moving along…

Remember that the free radicals and reactive oxygen species are produced by normal cellular functions, and most are dispensed with by the body's own natural defenses. Remember superoxide dismutase and catalase?

The uncontrolled radicals, however, react with proteins, lipids and DNA to cause significant molecular damage and aging.

When our astaxanthin molecule reaches an individual cell, and we'll get to transport later, it is able to incorporate into both the cell membrane and the mitochondrial membrane. The molecule inserts itself directly into the lipid bilayers, and spans the entire membrane.

Called a transmembrane orientation, this prime location allows the molecule to perform its magic in several subcellular components. As a direct result,

Location, Location, Location! ▶

astaxanthin is a far more potent free radical scavenger (ROS) than its molecular cousins. It is 200 times that of the other polyphenols, 150x anthocyanin, 75x alpha lipoic acid, 550x greater than vitamin E, 54x greater than Beta carotene, 6000x greater than Vitamin C, and 800x that of Coenzyme Q.[3]

When antioxidant capacities are compared, the results are basically the same. Astaxanthin is 10x greater than lutein and zeaxanthin, 14x greater than vitamin E, 54x greater than B-Carotene, 65x greater than Vitamin C and 100x greater in antioxidant activity than alpha tocopherol. Astaxanthin is simply more powerful than its competitors. Astaxanthin is quite unique; it can either accept or donate protons, but unlike many other substances, it does not itself become a pro-oxidant.

• •

"Astaxanthin has been shown to be one of the most effective antioxidants against lipid perioxidation and oxidative stress in in vivo and in vitro systems."[4]

• •

Therefore, any potential damage inflicted by the escapee free radicals is significantly reduced. As an interesting example of this, a study was done to measure the effects of astaxanthin on normal women and their DNA.

• •

Before I explain the study, it is cool to note that DNA damage can actually be measured. Specifically, we quantify the amount of 8-hydroxy-2- deoxyguanosine in the plasma.

• •

Unfortunately, constant DNA damage is a fact, and at least knowledge is empowering; thus, we can start doing something about it. Anyway, in 2010, a study looked at healthy 21.5 year old women (on average) that took placebo, 2 mg or 8 mg/day of astaxanthin for 8 weeks. Remarkably, both doses of astaxanthin significantly lowered the rate of DNA breakdown.[5] One of the interesting take-home messages here is that even people in their twenties are experiencing measurable DNA damage. They are already aging, they just don't know it.

Seeking more evidence of astaxanthin's power to combat free radicals, eyeball tissues in diabetic rats were examined for evidence of hyperglycemic induced, oxidative stress damage and its reversibility. Not only do high glucose levels increase the production of free oxygen radicals, it causes the depletion of cellular antioxidant defense capacities. Not unexpectedly, significant damage to the retina and surrounding eye tissues was noted in the control group. By comparison, the addition of astaxanthin to their diet, at a variety of concentrations, was extremely beneficial.

• •

"Ocular tissue from AST-treated rats had significantly reduced levels of oxidative stress mediators (8-8-hydroxy-2- deoxyguanosine, nitrotryosine, and acrolein) and inflammatory mediators....and increased levels of antioxidant enzymes..."[6]

• •

Thus, it was clearly demonstrated that the addition of astaxanthin had a protective effect and helped to preserve the retinal architecture and function of the ocular tissues.

• •

"Astaxanthin prevents cancer initiation by alleviating DNA oxidative damage."[3]

"AST is well known as a powerful free radical scavenger and an excellent anti-inflammatory agent that suppresses pro inflammatory cytokine and chemokine expression."[6]

"It is well worth mentioning that astaxanthin can act as a safeguard against oxidative damage through various mechanisms, by quenching of singlet oxygen, scavenging of radicals, inhibiting lipid preoccupation, and regulating gene expression related to oxidative stress."[7]

• •

How about oxidative stress in people?

Overweight or obese people are thought to be especially vulnerable to oxidative stress, and thus make good test subjects. To examine this, a study in 2011 measured markers of stress, (malondialdehyde and isoprostanes), and markers of antioxidant capacity, (superoxide dismutase and total antioxidant capacity).

As anticipated, the untreated obese population had higher stress markers and lower antioxidant capacity than normal weight people. After three weeks of astaxanthin therapy in the obese population, remarkably, all of the oxidative and stress markers and measures normalized; pretty impressive, especially after only a couple of weeks.[8]

In addition to possessing its own inherent antioxidant activity, astaxanthin also stimulates the bodies own defenses and increases the cellular levels of catalase, superoxide dismutase and peroxidase. At least this is known to occur in rats and rabbits.

Still working it out when it comes to people ▶

If you recall from the section on mitochondria, protecting the organelles from free radical damage is of the utmost importance.

• •

"Astaxanthin is not only able to protect against free radicals itself, it also stimulates production of the antioxidant enzymes catalase, superoxide disputes, and peroxidase."[2]

As noted by Wu in 2015, AST can act as a safeguard through a variety of mechanisms, by "quenching of singlet oxygen, scavenging of radicals, inhibiting lipid preoccupation and regulating gene expression related to oxidative stress."[7]

• •

To reinforce the idea that astaxanthin is good for your mitochondria, I offer even more evidence.

Yes, the cute little dogs! ▶

Unfortunately, studies on the effects of astaxanthin specifically looking at mitochondria are somewhat uncommon. There is however, a great study with beagles.[15]

Both young beagles and old beagles were given astaxanthin for sixteen weeks and a few things were uncovered.

First, not unexpectedly, the astaxanthin suppressed DNA damage; a lot in old dogs, a little in young dogs. Secondly, the mitochondrial mass increased in the geriatric dogs. Lastly, astaxanthin increased the ATP or energy production 12-14% in both the old and the young. So, it seems that the astaxanthin truly is beneficial to mitochondria.

Immune Systems / Security: Anti-inflammatory

The evidence for this quality is pretty substantial, and we will examine it from the cellular level up.

In 2012[9], a human cell line was bathed in astaxanthin in a warm and happy laboratory. The magical substance inhibited ROS-induced activation of NF-$\kappa\beta$, which then suppressed the production of IL-1β, IL-6 and TNF-α. If you remember from the inflammation chapter, these cytokines are able to inflict significant damage both locally and systemically. Limitation of this pathway is therefore a good thing.

To further support this, human microglial brain cells, also in a warm comfy environment, i.e., a cell culture, were disturbed by the addition of LPS (lipopolysacharide) which incites the production of inflammatory factors, especially IL-6. In this 2010 study,[10] the addition of astaxanthin to the culture medium suppressed production of IL-6 and NF-$\kappa\beta$.

Convinced that isolated cells benefited from astaxanthin, we turn our interests to actual mammals. Knowing that diabetes can wreak havoc on the entire body, but especially the brain, researchers set out to see if astaxanthin could be of any practical use in this arena. In a rat brain study, scientists replicated the diabetic scenario and then tried to improve the rats outcomes.

Actually they sacrificed the rats in the end, so their outcome was terrible regardless

After treatment with astaxanthin for 5 days, the neurocognitive skills of the diabetic rats were actually better than the non-diabetics. Researchers then looked at the actual brains of the diabetic, astaxanthin treated rats. Remarkably, the inflammatory markers, NF-$\kappa\beta$, TNF-α, IL-1B and IL-6, in the cerebral cortex and hippocampus were much improved. As an additional benefit, the astaxanthin also seemed to help control the blood sugar of the diabetic rats.[11]

In another very cool brain study, more rats were pretreated with astaxanthin and then inflicted with a subarachnoid hemorrhage.[12] Normally, blood on the brain is extremely inflammatory. As a side note, this is why people with subarachnoid hemorrhages have a high incidence of seizures. In this case, the supplement was found to reduce neutrophil infiltration, suppress activity of NF-κβ, and decrease IL-1β, TNF and ICAM-1(Intercellular adhesion molecule). Overall, the treatment dramatically reversed brain inflammation. As a result, there was reduced secondary brain injury, a reduction in neuronal degeneration, protection of the blood-brain barrier, limited cerebral edema and brain function was preserved.

Researchers love astaxanthin; they love torturing rats and they love saving brains. As a result, there is a plethora of additional research confirming the protective effect of the supplement on the rat brain. Therefore, I will sum up the take-home message.

Astaxanthin is able to cross the blood brain barrier, enter into neural tissue and work its magic through a multitude of properties.

• •

"Astaxanthin inhibits cyclooxygenase 2 (COX 2) enzyme activities, which are related with many diseases, such as osteoarthritis, rheumatoid arthritis, dysmenorrhea and acute pain."[3]

"Astaxanthin affects not only the COX 2 signaling pathway but also multiple cytokines, like nitric oxide, interleukin 1-β, prostaglandin E2, C-Reactive Protein (CRP), NF-κβ and TNF-α."[3]

• •

The next step in examining inflammation is looking at the granddaddy of all inflammation; sepsis. Sepsis is a full body phenomena whereby inflammation from an inciting factor causes damage systemically. It is a potentially life-threatening complication whereby chemicals that are released into the bloodstream to fight the infection trigger inflammatory responses throughout the body and cause more harm than good. Signs of sepsis usually include a very low blood pressure, swelling from dysfunctional capillaries, failure of multiple organ systems and very frequently, death. Generally speaking, sepsis is detrimental.

To test the protective effects of astaxanthin, rats were given a relatively high dose for 7 days, and then subjected to a procedure that induced sepsis. Compared to those rats without the treatment, the astaxanthin reduced the systemic inflammatory response (lower TNF, IL-1β, IL-6), alleviated organ injury, reduced peritoneal bacterial load, and improved survival of the rats. You may not care about the life of these little septic rats, but you may care if you ever find yourself in an ICU with a similar problem.[13]

Immune System / Security: Increase in Immunity

(Technically this should be in the same section as above, but it seemed different enough, I thought it needed its own space)

All right, astaxanthin seems to be effective at scavenging evil substances, but can it enhance the bodies own ability to fight infection? Absolutely.

In the same 2010 study demonstrating that astaxanthin could reduce DNA damage in young women, the study also noted an increased activity of natural killer cell cytotoxicity as well as increasing total T and B cell populations.[15]

I won't bore you with any more rat studies. But these are the general findings:

- Astaxanthin activates T-cells and can inhibit autoimmune reactions in rats.[3]
- IgG and IgM increases in cats and dogs.[14]

Meanwhile, in humans, our mucosal immune system is designed to defend against pathogens on mucosal surfaces such as in the gastrointestinal tract or respiratory tree. Leading this defensive arsenal are IgA molecules that attach themselves to threatening microorganisms and facilitate their elimination. As with everything good in the body, IgA secretion decreases with age. It also decreases with physiological and physical stress, nutritional deficiencies and intensive physical exertion. The good news is that astaxanthin can return these levels to normal.

Based on the properties that we have reviewed, it becomes quite clear that astaxanthin would have a positive effect on diseases associated with aging.

This is especially true for cardiovascular diseases. In many laboratory animals, astaxanthin was shown to lower systolic blood pressure, improve heart function, and helped prevent atherosclerosis and strokes.

In fact, many of the adjuvants we are going to review are beneficial in preventing and even treating cardiovascular disease. This is almost a baseline requirement for delaying aging, but every substance also does something unusual or special, and astaxanthin is a prime example. In particular, it is known to help with vision, skin, and even fitness.

Eyes

Of the many markers of age that every person faces is the need for reading glasses. Somewhere in the 40's or early 50's, this issue becomes seemingly unavoidable. We have all been out to a restaurant where someone borrows someone else's glasses. It may be the husband, the wife or the parents, but inevitably, a younger person ends up reading the bill or the credit card receipt.

The eye doctors tell me that this phenomena, presbyopia, is unpreventable; falling into the same category of general aging. In fact, before now, I had never read nor heard about anything that could help.

Why does this happen? First, it has nothing to do with being near or far sighted, which is an issue with eyeball shape. Presbyopia is related to the inherent flexibility of the lens inside the eye. In order to focus, the lens must change shape to accommodate close up vision. As the body ages, this lens, as well as the muscles around it, get stiffer and less elastic such that it becomes increasingly more difficult to focus.

But why does this happen? Because our eyes are victims of extreme stress without any inherent bailout mechanisms. More radiation and light penetrate eye tissues than any other, and the lens in the eye has very little blood flow. The lens does have antioxidant enzymes, but they of course decline with age. Therefore the lens experiences excessive and cumulative stress, with a reduced ability to self heal. Consequently, it is not too difficult to understand why vision fails in almost everyone at about the same period of time.

The retina is also a very stressed component of the eye. Like the lens, the retina is constantly pummeled with damaging radiation that creates very high levels of free radicals and DNA damage. Over time, this can lead to macular degeneration and blindness.

• •

> *The Japanese, however, love astaxanthin (almost as much as Russians love carnosine, as we will soon see), and are responsible for most of the vision and skin research. We owe a great deal of thanks to the Japanese in this area.*

• •

Astaxanthin to the rescue.

In 2009, Japanese researchers administered 6 mg daily to middle-aged people (46-65) for one month. Remarkably, 60% of the subjects had visual improvements, especially in the categories of "difficulty to see near objects," "eye strain" and "blurred vision."[16]

• •

> *"The retina contains high levels of unsaturated fatty acids and oxygen supply. The singlet oxygen is generated in the retina upon high-energy light illumination. ...Recent studies indicated that astaxanthin can pass through the blood-brain barrier and prevent retina cell oxidation."[3]*

• •

In a separate study, a combination of lutein, zeaxanthin and astaxanthin over the course of two years proved to provide stabilization and even improvement in visual acuity, contrast sensitivity, and visual function for normal people.[17]

So, our vision is eventually going to get worse, but at least now we can delay the process.

Skin

Skin should just be another organ; it is a protective cover that shields us from the brutal environment in which we live. It blocks radiation, repels chemicals, and defends against pathogens while retaining moisture and defining our boundaries.

Skin, however, is so much more than this; it can even define who we are. It denotes race. It determines who is attractive and who is not. It has even become a canvas for artists to decorate.

For our conversation however, skin is the outermost visual representation of aging because this is what we see in the mirror, and when we look at other people. We can't see the internal markers of aging, but we can see our skin sag. We see discoloration. Over time, the face gets creased, the hands get spots, and crows feet develop.

It's what keeps the plastic surgeons in business!

In reality, our skin really is just another organ. The good news however, is that because it's on the outside, we can treat it in two ways. We can apply corrective remedies topically, and we can take them internally.

What does this mean for astaxanthin? It turns out that one of the coolest things astaxanthin does is block damage to the skin from the environment, especially radiation.

In human cell lines, especially skin fibroblasts and melanocytes, astaxanthin was shown to reduce DNA damage that was precipitated by UVA radiation. Remember that UVA radiation causes damage by creating free radicals that then destroy DNA.

Given, most of the studies with skin cells and radiation have been done in isolated cells sitting in a dish, but this effect applies to real people as well. It thus turns out that astaxanthin can actually block sun damage from the inside. It can't block all the DNA damage, so don't throw away the sunscreen, but it can block a significant portion.[18]

The first ever internal sunblock... Pretty amazing!

Astaxanthin doesn't just prevent skin damage, it turns out it can actually improve it. Again, the Japanese are on the ball here. In 2011, 30 healthy Japanese women ranging in age from 20 to 55 used astaxanthin both as a supplement (6 mg) and as a topical cream for 2 months. The women were thrilled; there was definitive skin improvement in crows feet, age spot size, elasticity, skin texture, and the moisture content of corneocytes.[19]

In essence, study after study have proclaimed the beautifying effects of astaxanthin. What could be better?

Fitness

As a side trip in the anti-aging journey, we are going to talk about physical exercise for a minute. As I have said previously, this is not a lecture on why anyone should exercise. I can, however, tell you why astaxanthin can help you to exercise.

At the heart of it, physical activity is essentially any movement that raises the heart rate and moves the muscles. To accomplish this, the requirement for oxygen and energy of course, goes up. Thus, we are requiring the mitochondria to increase production. Harder working mitochondria, as we are now aware, leads to an increase in free radicals and oxidative stress, and thus the potential for increased cellular and DNA damage. Aerobic exercise is actually associated with an increase of up to 80 fold higher volume of oxygen, so this concern is quite valid.

Academic couch potatoes use this as an excuse to avoid exercise entirely

Astaxanthin, taken on a chronic basis, can actually prevent this excess production of free radicals and make it safe to exercise.

To confirm this, we return to our lab animals. And, in the never ending challenge to find more ways to torture small mammals, young astaxanthin-laden mice were put on a treadmill. While control mice demonstrated the standard amount of protein and DNA damage, the astaxanthin mice did not.[20]

In an even more torturous study, astaxanthin fed rats were forced to swim. Not unexpectedly, these rats demonstrated decreased levels of oxidative stress, and increased plasma antioxidant capacity as compared to the controls.

Even more interesting, the astaxanthin rats swam longer. In what they called a 'forced swimming activity,' the rats were encouraged to swim until they almost drown, (submerged and unresponsive for 3-5 seconds) at which time they were rescued and then decapitated. Torture methods aside, the astaxanthin rats swam 29% longer. That is really remarkable if you think about it. An almost 30% increase in exercise capacity is unheard of in the world of exercise improvements.[21]

Does it work in humans? This is actually really hard to say. One study in 17 to 19-year-old boys given astaxanthin for six months showed improvements in some strength and endurance activities, but not all.[8] Studies in trained athletes have been contradictory regarding actual physical improvement. Perhaps they should have tried the 'forced swimming activity.'

I'm kidding! ▶

As an interesting aside, even if our maximal physical capacity does not improve with astaxanthin, the linear swimming velocity of sperm in infertile men does. Given 16 mg/day for three months to men that were clinically infertile, the pregnancy rate rose to 50% over the course of the study versus 10.5% in the control group.

Back to the molecule itself, astaxanthin exists as a fat soluble compound. Not that that really matters, except that it follows the same intestinal absorption path as dietary fat. In fact, dietary oils can enhance absorption, while the absence of bile or malfunction of lipid absorption can reduce absorption (Don't take a fat blocker with this if you're on a diet). Therefore, you are better off if you take it with food in terms of absorption. Oddly, it is 40% less bioavailable in smokers.

But no one reading this probably smokes, so it really doesn't matter. ▶

Once ingested, astaxanthin gets absorbed into the bloodstream and taken to the liver where it is repackaged into lipoproteins and transported around the body (both as LDL and HDL). Where does it go? Hard to say in people, but in rats it accumulates in viscera such as the spleen, kidneys, adrenal glands and eyes. Accumulation and elimination in the skin appears to be much slower, but it does occur.

Pharmacodynamic data indicate that a single 10 mg dose in a human can persist in the blood for 24 hours, while a 100 mg dose can last up to 76 hours. Doses as low as 1 mg can increase blood levels if taken daily for up to 4 weeks.[3]

How much do you need? Again, hard to say.

It's possible they turned a little red though! ▶

Animals have been given well over 120 mg/day without any ill effects.

In humans, it has been tested for acute toxicity, mutagenicity, teratogenicity, embryo toxicity and reproductive toxicity and no issues have been uncovered.

If you want to consume it naturally, I recommend the fish. Sockeye salmon has the highest content, ranging from 26-38 mg/kg.[2] Farmed Atlantic salmon has a measly 6-8 mg/kg by comparison.

Doses in pill form range anywhere from 1 to 40 mg/day; but the vast majority are in the 2 - 12 mg range.

The popularity of astaxanthin is growing almost exponentially. In fact, as of 2014, patent applications for various uses were piling up with a wide range of uses. These have been identified as "preventing bacterial infection, inflammation, vascular failure, cancer, cardiovascular diseases, inhibiting lipid preoccupation, reducing cell damage and body fat, and improving brain function and skin thickness."[2]

So, this colorful, omnipresent and omni-helpful yogi can only serve you well. He will diminish your stress, protect your DNA, smooth your wrinkles, clear your vision, and maybe even make you happier.

Kaufmann Number: 0.3.0.0.2.0.0

CHAPTER 13:

NICOTINAMIDE ADENINE DINUCLEOTIDE

Because trust me, he's the type of friend you want! ▶ To better understand nicotinamide, we are first going to personify him and then befriend him.

"Nick," (not extremely clever, granted...but it will do), is more important than you can imagine, and a guy we would all love to hang out with. Picture Nick as a youthful, energetic kid that started working in the mailroom factory. He is ambitious, pleasant, extremely helpful and has made himself indispensable. Specifically, he will be carrying protons in the inner matrix of the mitochondria, but more about that later.

Nick proved to be a hard worker, and thus in addition to his mailroom responsibilities, he was promoted as a repairman to work in the head office, or nucleus. Again, more specifically, he works in DNA repair mechanisms.

Doing a great job there, he was once again promoted. This time he was to be on the communication team that transmits information from the nucleus to the mitochondria.

As if poor Nick wasn't busy enough, he was then handed perhaps the biggest responsibility yet. Nick was adopted into the sirtuin family, where he became absolutely indispensable. In fact, he became a necessary co-factor in all of their dealings. This means that without Nick, the vast anti-aging aspects of the sirtuin family would not function at all. In this role, Nick helps to control circadian rhythms, modulates cellular senescence, protects nerves against traumatic injury and can even modulate aging.

So, our friend Nick has become a multi-departmental supervisor while still maintaining his role as simple mailroom carrier. In short, Nick is the perfect employee; he does it all; but, like all very diligent and multifunctional employees, when they get tired or stretched too thin, things begin to deteriorate.

The same fate holds for our real molecule of nicotinamide. Over time, we require more and more of it, while, as the overwhelming theme of this book has illustrated, the availability actually drops. Like pushing our friend Nick too far, we have come to demand too much of a single substance, and the inevitable shortage leads to a cellular crisis. What we see with time and reduced nicotinamide is failed mitochondria, failed intracellular communication, increased DNA failure and advanced aging.

The good news is that, of course, this is fixable. But, let's start from the beginning so that all of this makes sense.

Nicotinamide adenine dinucleotide (NAD) consists of two nucleotides joined together by their phosphate groups. One nucleotide contains an adenine base, the other a nicotinamide; hence the name.

NAD is made naturally in the body, beginning with the amino acid tryptophan. Eight steps later, it is converted into our usable substance. As this process is slow and frequently cannot keep up with demand, the body also utilizes a salvage pathway, whereby the used NAD can be repaired, or chemically altered, such that it is usable once again.

For reasons that will be discussed shortly, the demand for NAD rises with age, and the more efficient salvage pathway becomes more important than the slower, de novo production. As well, it has been more recently discovered that there are several nicotinamide-ish intermediates that can be converted to usable NAD. Examples include various forms of the vitamin B3, such as nicotinic acid, straight nicotinamide and nicotinamide ribosome that are all present in our diet.

While a relative lack of NAD becomes apparent with age (if you know what to look for), a more significant deficiency is responsible for the disease of Pellagra. Secondary to a poor diet, and thus the vitamin deficiency, Pellagra is generally noted by the 4 D's: diarrhea, dermatitis, dementia and death. A lack of NAD, therefore is clearly not a good thing. The cure for years, at least in the deep south, was the drinking of cow's milk. They were not aware of it until 1937, but it turns out that the raw milk contained reasonable amounts of nicotinamide (60% as straight Nicotinamide, 40% as Nicotinamide riboside) and thus could reverse the deficiency.[1]

As we are now aware, Nick has innumerable roles in our factory. Let's look at them from the ground up.

Mitochondria / Energy systems: Activities in the Mitochondria

The first of the responsibilities we mentioned earlier was as a delivery boy in the mail room. On a cellular level, this translates into transporting electrons and protons in the mitochondria. If you recall from the introductory chapters, the mitochondria has an inner and an outer membrane. By pumping electrons "up hill" along the electron transport chain in the inner membrane, an energy gradient is created that ultimately creates ATP. NAD is a key participant in that it can carry electrons. Thus, nicotinamide gets continuously converted back and forth from NAD+ to NADH.

In more science terms, NAD+ is called an oxidizing agent as it can accept electrons from other molecules and then become reduced to NADH. The opposite reaction is then able to donate or pass the electrons elsewhere, and regenerate the NAD+.

$$NAD+ + H+ + 2e- \Longleftrightarrow NADH$$

Under-standing the in and outs falls into geek territory so don't worry about it!

• •

"Although the redox role of NAD+ is well established, there is renewed interest in NAD+ metabolism due to recent evidence showing that NAD+ regulates diverse pathways including those controlling lifespan."[2,3]

• •

There are specific ratios of NAD+ to NADH within the cellular compartments that maximize energy efficiency, but that goes beyond the scope of this discussion. It is important to note though, that as NAD levels decline with age, the ratios and thus energy production dwindles as well.

Thus, the take-home message here is that without NAD, energy becomes a very scarce resource.

Pathways: Obligate Sirtuin Co-Factor

Another family of genes and proteins that are dependent on NAD is the SIRTUIN clan. As we discussed earlier, these genes are highly correlated with health and longevity. In these biochemical processes, NAD serves as a necessary co-factor. This means that once again, the NAD molecule gets deconstructed and consumed.

We know that sirtuin activity declines with age, but recent evidence suggests that the decline in NAD actually is responsible for the loss of sirtuin activity over time. It turns out that the quantity of available NAD can in fact control the activity of sirtuins.

As a quick review, the sirtuins, numbered 1-7 in mammals, are a family of NAD-dependent (obviously) lysine modifying amylases that control responses to exercise and diet. SIRT1 expression, the first and most studied, is known to extend lifespan and overexpression of such has positive health benefits. These are known to include protection from metabolic decline, cardiovascular disease, cancer and neurodegeneration. Sirtuin activation also increases the antioxidant pathways (SOD2), facilitates DNA repairs and enhances metabolic efficiency.[4]

To further support the importance of the sirtuins, a reduction in SIRT1 activity down regulates almost all the things that are beneficial. Mitochondrial biogenesis, oxidative metabolism, and antioxidant defenses are diminished and there is a general decline in mitochondrial function.

• •

> *"Since cellular NAD+ levels are limiting for sirtuin activity, boosting its level is a powerful means to activate sirtuins as a potential therapy for mitochondrial, often age-related, diseases....Indeed, supplying excess precursors... boosts NAD+ levels, activates sirtuins and promotes healthy aging."[5]*

• •

An interesting byproduct of the association of NAD with the sirtuins is the intracellular communication between the nucleus and the mitochondria. There exists something called an OXPHOS or oxidative phosphorylation system, whereby the nucleus controls the mitochondria. This system is constructed of subunits that are partly manufactured in the nucleus, and partly in the mitochondria. The nuclear-produced subunits are controlled by the sirtuins, which in turn is controlled by the available NAD. Therefore, when there is low NAD in the nucleus, the nucleus essentially tells the mitochondria to stop energy production.

Quality Control: DNA Repair Mechanisms

As we have noted already, aging is characterized by increases in the amount of DNA damage. From free radicals to simple replication errors, over time, DNA takes a beating. The good news, of course, is that the cell is capable of fixing most of these problems. If you recall from the Maintenance or Quality Control chapter, the job of DNA repair is assigned to a family of genes and associated proteins called PARPs, short for poly-ADP-ribose polymerase. PARPs are responsible for the recognition of DNA damage and then directing its repair.

Of note, the measurable activity of PARPs in white blood cells correlates extremely well with the maximum lifespan in innumerable mammalian species, including rats, guinea pigs, rabbits, sheep, elephants and people. Thus, repair of DNA is an absolutely necessary activity to promote health and longevity.

Once the PARPs locate an error in the DNA, they activate the appropriate repair system, i.e., Base excision repair or Nucleotide excision repair for example, and then acquire the materials necessary for the actual reconstruction. Just as a brick layer can only fix a hole in a wall if he has a pile of bricks, PARPs turn to NAD as a raw material.

In this instance, NAD is referred to as a co-substrate, but in reality, the molecule is cleaved apart and pieces of it are literally placed into the DNA to fix the hole. Thus, the molecule is not recycled as it is in the mitochondria, but it is completely consumed.

Thus, the older one gets and the more DNA damage that accrues, the more active PARPs become and the more NAD is required. As I mentioned in an earlier chapter, PARPs are considered voracious scavengers of NAD.

• •

> *"PARP1 utilizes NAD as a substrate and participates in DNA-base excision repair, DNA damage signaling, regulation of genomic function, transcription and proteasomal functions. However, PARP1 depletes intracellular NAD, and therefore, leads to cell death by necrosis."[6]*

• •

Thus it is clear that NAD has a HUGE role in cellular metabolism and energy production as a whole. Our problem starts in the fact that (1) our NAD levels drop with age, and (2) our body's requirements for NAD rise.

Why does NAD decline with age? We really don't know for sure. Murphy's Law, perhaps? The reality is that it is a combination of several things, including a decline in production and an increase in utilization.

• •

"Aging also has a significant impact on NAD biosynthesis at the cellular and organismal level, resulting in reduced NAD levels in human cells and rodents."[7]

• •

We know that the main enzyme responsible for producing NAD from its immediate precursor, NAMPT aka nicotinamide phosphoribosyl-transferase, declines with age. We also know that inflammation, or especially Tumor necrosis factor-α (TNF-α), and oxidative stress suppress NAMPT. Therefore NAD levels decline as stress and inflammatory factors increase. So, overall, we produce less NAD with age.

• •

"Exercise training interestingly increases the activity of NAMPT, increasing levels of NAD and boosting your energy."[8]

• •

We also require increasing amounts. The NAD utilized for DNA repair, for example, increases with age. As well, as we strive to maintain our youthful sirtuin-controlled genes, we need to stabilize circadian rhythms, and we require energy. Thus, a tug-of-war ensues over the allocation of NAD.

The choice of where the body invests the declining resource determines which system will fail first. Stealing NAD from the mitochondria will lead to reduced energy levels. Displacing it from the DNA repair system will lead to cancer. Turning off the sirtuins leads to accelerated aging. Regardless of what the body chooses, we lose.

The good news, of course, is that we can do something about this. Much like treating Pellagra, we can replenish our stores. How do we know this? Lots of measurements and the torturing of small rodents. I'm not going to bore you with study after study showing that augmentation with a NAD precursor leads to an increase in NAD, you are just going to have

It just does! ▶ to believe me.

● ●

"NAD+ repletion improves mitochondrial and stem cell function and enhances life span in mice."[9]

"Partial reversal of skeletal muscle aging by restoration of normal NAD+ levels..."[10]

● ●

The real question, however, is which one to choose?

As there are many precursors to NAD, different researchers have taken different paths to determine how best to augment the levels. Studies have examined the effects of additional straight nicotinamide, nicotinic acid and nicotinamide riboside. Nicotinic acid, also called Niacin, has been used for years to treat Pellagra and even hyperlipidemia. The high doses required typically could cause flushing, but are now made in a slow-release form and the side effect is diminished.

Not to be confused with Nicotine... Smoking definitely does not help!

High doses of straight nicotinamide meanwhile, have been shown to decrease levels of sirtuins and even PARPs, leading to a decline in cellular function. It can also cause liver toxicity.[11] This, therefore, is not a great option.

Nicotinamide riboside (NR) seems to be the winner thus far, and in fact many very brilliant scientists are staking their reputations and pocket books on it. NR can be converted to usable NAD in 2 metabolic steps.[11] It turns out this formulation is stable, easy to produce and reasonably inexpensive.

So, is NR commercially available? Of course it is, but it is only produced by one company, Chromadex. This publicly traded company acquired the intellectual property on the uses and synthesis of NR from Dartmouth College, Cornell and Washington University and began distributing NR under the name Niagen in 2013. Chromadex holds five US patents as well as several international patents on the formulation.

In 2015, the company started the ball rolling by demonstrating that a single dose of NR could in fact increase the level of NAD in the human body. Presently, (while I'm writing this in 2016) a second study is underway to examine the health benefits in adults (40 to 60 years of age) taking the supplement for 8 consecutive weeks.

The folks at Chromadex are not the only ones to believe heavily in the effects of NR. A second company, Elysium health, has the same belief. The co-founder, Dr. Lenny Guarantee is/was a professor at MIT for 35 years with a PhD from Harvard, and sits with six Nobel Laureates on the advisory board. The point here, is if you don't believe me, all of these incredible bright humans probably are not wrong. Regardless, this company makes one product, called Basis, which has two ingredients. One of these is, of course, NR.

In any event, as researchers continue to study the effects of increasing NAD, more and more positive effects are being discovered. Scientists have also discovered some very interesting little quirks of NAD.

One of my favorites of these interesting attributes revolves around hearing loss from loud noises. Intense noise exposure generally causes a decline in hearing by inducing degeneration of the spiral ganglion nerves that innervate cochlear hair cells. More simply, loud noise kills the nerves in your ears. Interestingly, NR given to mice activates a SIRT3 pathway that reduces the degeneration of these nerves and thus preserves their hearing.[12]

• •

"Administration of NR, even after noise exposure, prevents noise induced hearing loss and spiral ganglia neurite degeneration."[12]

• •

In other words, a little NR can save your hearing from that ridiculously loud rock concert.

As I stated in the beginning, Nick is pretty impressive; but you don't really notice him until he's no longer there.

Kaufmann Number: 0.3.3.3.0.0.0

CHAPTER 14:

CURCUMIN

The story of curcumin is a long and very old one. This semi-ephemeral substance has been around for over five thousand years, and has traveled the globe bringing health and well-being to people everywhere; and yet, it is vastly under-appreciated... at least by western civilizations.

The substance can be traced to its early use in Vedic India four thousand years ago, where it was used both as a spice and in religious ceremonies. It arrived in China somewhere near 700 AD and then East Africa by 800 AD. Curcumin was praised by Avicenna, a Persian Physician, in a famous medieval medical text called "The Canon" (his name was actually Abu Ali al Husain Ebn Abdullah Ebn Sina; 980-1037 AD) who was considered to be the most learned and influential physician at the time. Curcumin was then smuggled to Europe by Marco Polo in 1280. In Sanskrit, there are no less than fifty-three different names for the substance, each representing a different quality. Clearly, the value of this substance was recognized by one civilization after another, adapted and then utilized to fulfill their needs.

As it spread, curcumin became many things to many people. It is a spice, essential in Asian cooking. In fact, it is a key ingredient in many dishes from

India, Nepal, South Africa, Vietnam, Cambodia, Indonesia, and Thailand. It adds flavor and color, as well as serving as a food preservative.

Worldwide, it is used in religious ceremonies and it is even worn as an amulet in southern Indian to protect against evil spirits. For Buddhist monks, the bright yellow dye colors their traditional clothing.

In Indian and Chinese medicine, it has been used for innumerable maladies, including jaundice or excessive flatulence. It is an appetite suppressant and aids in digestion. It treats standard aches and pains, many types of infections and skin lesions, and even lung diseases.

In Pakistan, it is considered an anti-inflammatory. In Afghanistan, it is an anti-septic. In Bangladesh and India, it is believed to make the skin glow.

Curcumin, it seems, is omnipotent yet surprisingly benign. Over the thousands of years, people have trialled it for almost everything, making it perhaps the most tested adjuvant available ever. If there was anything that might benefit from its use, someone in some millennia probably discovered it. As well, if curcumin did not deliver as expected, it would have been abandoned long ago.

So, what exactly is this phenomenal substance? Curcumin is one of the active molecules from the spice turmeric. Turmeric, meanwhile, comes from the roots or the rhizomes of *Curcuma longa*. This herbaceous, perennial plant belongs in the ginger family, *Zingiberaceae*, and grows in wet regions where the temperature is between 68 to 86 degrees F. Most turmeric is grown in India, and they also consume 80% of it.

To begin the processing, the root or rhizome is first boiled or steamed. Once upon a time, this root was then placed in water, and covered with leaves and cow dung. Apparently ammonia in the cow feces reacted with the rhizome to finish the process. Clearly, this is not done any more, but kudos to the person that invented the process. Today, the rhizomes are boiled in alkaline water and then dried.

Once processed, turmeric becomes a bright yellow powder and is known as Indian Saffron; it is what gives curry and Ethiopian rice its distinctive color. It is described as being "distinctly earthly, slightly bitter, slightly hot peppery flavor with a mustardy smell" by Wikipedia.

AKA the Millenial's encyclopedia ▶

Interestingly, if turmeric gets exposed to acid, it turns bright red. Because of this quality, it can and was used as a pH detector prior to the advent of litmus paper.

Turmeric, the base root, contains a wide variety of difficult to pronounce phytochemicals in addition to curcumin, including demethoxycurcumin, bisdemethoxycurcumin, zingiberene, curcumenol, eugenol, and a bunch of others that need not be listed. Overall, there are about 100 of them, but it is the curcumin that grants the substance its magnificent color and its therapeutic effects. Unfortunately, curcumin only constitutes between 3 to 5% of the turmeric, and thus you require a lot of turmeric to get even a little curcumin.

Identified in 1910, the scientific or formal name of curcumin is actually diferuloylmethane. Apparently not as catchy, the name never caught on.

Therefore, curcumin is our actual hero in this story. He is not a true hero in the traditional sense, but he should be. He has been around for thousands of years quietly aiding humanity, he has traveled from civilization to civilization and solved innumerable problems plaguing mankind, and he has done this with very little fanfare.

Our folk hero, however, has recently left the confines of history and for the past several decades has been studied, scrutinized and dissected down to the molecular level; and, what I find incredibly amazing about the findings over the last 20 years is that curcumin has truly proven its worth. This magical substance really can do all that it is said to do and now, we know why!

Simply stated, curcumin is a free radical scavenger, an antioxidant and an anti-inflammatory. Secondary to these very potent qualities, it has far-reaching effects all over the body. Curcumin has proven to reduce the incidence of cancer, it can improve cognition and delays brain diseases. It reduces full body inflammation, and it can even reduce the amount of lipofuscin in your cells.

• •

"Curcumin has an unprecedented number of molecular targets. Due to these actions, curcumin can influence several conditions, among which cancer, neurodegeneration and aging are the most important."[1]

• •

But alas, too much too soon. One thing at a time.

Let's run the list:

DNA / Information systems: Epigenetics

Curcumin is also a part of the epigenetic diet, along with several other of our adjuvants.

But first, a quick DNA review...

The basic plan of DNA is a double helix, or spiraling ladder consisting of 4 base pairs. This double helix is then packaged by wrapping around an eight pack cluster of histones which helps to keep the DNA organized.

Regular genetics is the study of the actual base pair order and what it represents. The study of epigenetics is what is then added on. It turns out that on the DNA strands, at particular junctions, a methyl group has been attached. This methyl group acts as both a marker and a blocking agent; it controls which genes are being read and transcribed. In this way, proteins or enzymes that are not required are blocked from being produced.

In much the same manner, the histones get decorated with additions as well. These can be either methyl groups, acetyl groups or even phosphate groups. Regardless, this is another roadblock, preventing the DNA from being active.

When people are young, there are certain patterns of DNA and histone methylation. When we age, these patterns change. At one point, scientists tried to determine if the degree of methylation went up or down with age. Now we know that the absolute degree of methylation may not be consistent, but what changes is the pattern of methylation. In young DNA, the areas of methylation are very discrete and dense; i.e., heavy in some areas with very little in others. As we age, this pattern reverses. The methylation becomes more spread out throughout the DNA.

If you remember from the DNA chapter, sporadic changing of the DNA/ histone modification within an individual over time is called epigenetic drift. This accounts for the increasing differences in identical twins as they age. On the other hand, the common or anticipated epigenetic alterations that occur in almost everyone constitutes the basis for the epigenetic clock. Recall, as well, that there were substances that can mediate or minimize these changes.

What does this have to do with curcumin? Two things.

First, researchers have been looking for conditions that correlate with epigenetic drift. One of the clearest associations at this point is chronic inflammation. The more the body is inflamed over time, the more drift there appears to be. Clearly, curcumin reduces the magnitude of chronic inflammation, and thus can slow the deterioration of DNA.

Secondly, curcumin affects histone acetylation; it represses the addition of an acetyl group onto histone proteins. Specifically, it inhibits p300/CREB-specific acetyl transferase (another geeky detail). Therefore, it contributes to the control of DNA modification.[2] To be honest, I am assuming this is a good thing. I don't really know if anyone has determined exactly which histone complex should be acetylated or deacetylated, but as curcumin seems to be beneficial to us, I am assuming it works in a positive way. As well, it qualifies curcumin to be a part of the epigenetic diet.

Mitochondria / Energy systems: Anti-oxidant

The second key property of curcumin is as an antioxidant and free radical scavenger. Discovered around 1994, this is thought to be due to the Beta diketone in its structure.

• •

"Curcumin has been shown to have potent antioxidant activity that effectively scavenges ROS and inhibits lipid peroxidation."[3]

• •

Like many of the antioxidants, curcumin is highly lipophilic and can effectively permeate through cell walls and intercept free radicals both in the intracellular and cytoplasmic spaces. Curcumin is capable of combating many varieties of reactive species including the following: superoxide radicals, hydrogen peroxide, nitric oxide, and singlet oxygen.[4]

Curcumin apparently acts as both a direct free radical scavenger, and an indirect one. It enhances the production of the naturally occurring antioxidant enzymes, such as catalase, superoxide dismutase (SOD), glutathione peroxidase (GPx), glutathione reductase (GR), heme oxygenase-1 (OH-1), and glutathione S-transferase (GST). In essence, curcumin increases the total antioxidant capacity of the cell system.[4]

Pathways: Activates AMP Kinase.

Such an irrefutable argument, I know... ▶ How does it help the pathways? It just does!

In fact, curcuminoids increased the activation of AMP Kinase in liver cells in one study with 100,000 times the potency of metformin.[5]

To reinforce this point, I cite two studies:

In the first study, "the activation of AMPK signaling by curcumin was found to be involved in the anti-differentiation, anti-gluconeogenic, and anti-hepatic steatosis effect of curcumin."[6]

In the second, " ...reports demonstrated that curcumin can modulate activation of the 5'-AMP activated protein kinase (AMPK) signaling pathway, which is associated with aging-related vascular endothelial dysfunction in old mice."[7]

Immune system / Security

The inflammatory system, as we have discussed earlier, is a bimodal system. Early inflammation can be beneficial in terms of fighting off immediate infections. Chronic inflammation, however, becomes uncontrolled and is one of the prime components of aging and chronic disease. Chronic inflammation causes cellular stress, increased cardiovascular disease, brain damage, fibrosis of tissues, pain and innumerable other problems. There is a reason that anti-inflammatory medications are taken daily by millions of people every day.

I'm hoping this sounds vaguely familiar... ▶ The inflammatory tree is quite complex as we have seen as well. Near the very top of this chain is Tumor Necrosis Factor (TNF-α) and Nuclear Factor - kappa Beta (NF-κβ).

TNF gets activated by evils in the environment and subsequently activates NF-kB. These evils can include free radicals, radiation, carcinogens, ultraviolet light, tumor promotors, inflammatory cytokines, viruses, high glucose, fatty acids, and even psychological stress.

Once activated, NF-κβ gets translocated into the nucleus, where it initiates a cascade by turning on over 200 genes that further the inflammatory cycle. These include, but are not limited to, the inflammatory genes and resultant products such as cyclooxygenase-2 (COX-2), Lipo-oxygenase (LOX), cell adhesion molecules, C-reactive protein, IL-1β, IL-2, IL-5, IL-6, IL-8, 12 and 18.

While human studies are reasonably rare, there was an interesting study of 98 Iranian males that suffered from chronic and debilitating itching from exposure to sulphur mustard. Pruritus is generally a result of histamine release which is a result of the inflammatory pathway. After a month of oral curcumin treatment, there was a significant decline in the degree of itching.[8]

As it turns out, the real reason curcumin has such abilities is that it is a selective kinase inhibitor, and in this case, the activation of NF-κβ is blocked.

There are in fact many other detrimental cascades that are controlled by protein kinase enzymes, and curcumin can positively effect them. By inhibiting phosphorous kinase, curcumin controls all of the serine/threonine kinase pathways that control cell proliferation and even energy production.

More recently it was discovered that even above NF-κβ on the inflammatory pathway, TNF-α, which stimulates NF-κβ, is also blocked by curcumin. Therefore, curcumin blocks the very production of TNF at the gene level; the protein is not transcribed from the DNA, and thus even more of the inflammatory cascade is blocked.[2]

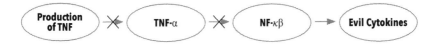

As a result, the top two tiers of the inflammatory cascade are essentially turned off or down, making it one of the most powerful anti-inflammatory agents available. Thus, it is possible to dispense with most, if not all, of the deleterious effects of the chronic inflammatory cycle.

• •

The list goes
on and on... ▶ *"How a single agent can possess these diverse effects has been an enigma over the years, both for basic scientists and clinicians. However, numerous lines of evidence have indicated curcumins ability in human participants to modulate multiple cell signaling molecules such as pro-inflammatory cytokines, apoptotic proteins, NFκβ, cyclooxygenase-2, STAT3, IKKB, MDA, CRP, GSH...."*[9]

• •

Therefore, over the millennia, curcumin has become a mainstay of treatment for any illness that ends in '-itis'. For example, ulcerative colitis, rheumatoid arthritis, pancreatitis, bronchitis, sinusitis, rhinitis, gingivitis, proctitis, and uveitis are all conditions associated with chronic inflammation. In fact there are probably about 200 '-itis' conditions that benefit from curcumin therapy.[2]

In real human studies, curcumin is thus transitioning from being considered an 'alternative medicine' to being a very practical medication. For example, in men undergoing hernia surgery, oral curcumin was able to reduce swelling, tenderness, and operative site pain.

Curcumin given to patients with rheumatoid arthritis (1200 mg/day) was effective in improving joint swelling, morning stiffness, and walking time.[10] After eight months of treatment, the ability to walk on a treadmill tripled, and serum markers for inflammation such as IL-1β, IL-6, and erythrocyte sedimentation rate were all significantly decreased.

In a comparative study of knee osteoarthritis, 1,500 mg/day of curcumin was equivalent to 1,200 mg of ibuprofen in terms of pain control. Of note, there were less gastrointestinal side effects with the curcumin.[11]

Significant improvements were also noted in studies looking at irritable bowel syndrome and inflammatory bowel diseases.

And avoiding
that is why
we're all
here! ▶ Realizing that quenching of inflammation may not seem very important, recall that the chronic state of inflammation contributes highly to the process of aging.

• •

"As low grade inflammation is believed to contribute substantially to aging, slowing aging, and postponing the onset of age-related diseases may be achieved by blocking NK-κβ dependent inflammation."[1]

• •

Chronic inflammation is also linked to cancer. Thus, it has been suggested that reducing inflammation can prevent some malignancies. Preclinical research, meaning in cell cultures but not humans themselves, have suggested that curcumin could be preventative against a number of cancers including colorectal, pancreatic, gastric, prostate, liver, multiple myeloma, lung, head and neck, breast and oral cancers.[9,10]

• •

"It is well understood that proinflammatory states are linked to tumor production."[10]

• •

Waste Management

As you may remember in the chapter on Waste Management, lipofuscin is the material that gets tucked away in the corner of the cell when it can't get recycled. This is a huge problem for long-lived cells, especially nerve cells in the brain.

One of the most amazing discoveries about curcumin is that it can actually reduce the amount of brain lipofuscin, as well as prevent cellular decline.

I find this so cool that I want to share some of the experimental details:

Curcumin was given to young, middle-aged and old rats for 3 months… and then their brains were examined, and compared to those that hadn't had the adjuvant. Several things were determined:

- Young brains have very little lipofuscin. (Not surprising) Old brains without curcumin have an abundance. On curcumin, middle-aged rats had way less than expected, about 1/3 that of the old rats. Treated old rats had about 2/3 that of untreated rats. Clearly, curcumin prevented some of the formation of lipofuscin. But remarkably, it was actually able to clean out some of the waste as well. It also showed that the earlier the treatment was started, the better off the result.

- Curcumin treatment prevented excessive damage to the mitochondria over time. The old, treated rat brains had significantly less structurally devastated organelles than the untreated old rats. As well, the curcumin treatment prevented the age-associated decline in most of the mitochondrial proteins including the electron transport chain complexes.

- As a result of the improved condition of the aging mitochondria, the resultant ATP or energy production was rescued. Specifically, in the old, untreated rats, ATP production was reduced by about half, (53.77%) as compared to the young rats. Treatment with curcumin rescued this and returned ATP production to 87% of normal.

Combination effect of waste products and anti-inflammatory quality: RAGE (receptor for AGEs) production blocked

In general, the presence of AGEs in the body stimulates the production of receptors for such on various cell walls (you may want to glance back at the chapter on Waste Management). Thus, the greater the quantities of AGEs, the greater the number of receptors. Activated receptors then precipitate the cascade of inflammatory factors leading to a host of negative consequences. Luckily, curcumin inhibits the gene expression for the receptors, blocking this negative relationship.[12] Therefore there are less receptors to start with. In addition, of course, curcumin can stave off whatever inflammation was precipitated in the first place. A double win.

Antimicrobial (This doesn't really help with the anti-aging process, but it's useful nonetheless)

Curcumin has a broad spectrum of antimicrobial activity including antibacterial, antiviral, anti-fungal and even antimalarial.[13]

The agent has proven to be active against common strains of human infection such as *Staph Aureus, Klebsiella Pneumonia, Staph Epidermis, E. Coli, Listeria Monocytogenes,* and even *Helicobacter pylori.* Realizing this list means very little to anyone outside of the medical world, these are extremely common bacteria that cause everyday skin infections, respiratory infections and stomach ulcers.

In addition, curcumin is synergistic with a variety of antibiotics including tetracycline, vancomycin, ampicillin, and even cefixime. Therefore, the dose of the more toxic antibiotic may be decreased if our adjuvant is used concomitantly.

Viruses, meanwhile, are quite challenging to treat and traditionally have been left to the world of vaccines and chicken soup. However, there is very solid evidence that curcumin has anti-influenza activity (the flu), works against human papilloma virus and coxsackie virus, and even exhibits some anti-HIV activity.

Realizing this is an extremely dry subject, the take-home message is that the ancient medics were correct yet again. Curcumin does have anti-septic properties. The argument however, is why use curcumin when we have more specialized therapies and specific treatments? I would counter that if one could prevent any of these infections or treat them very early, the potential side effects would be minimized as well as any downtime spent being sick. As well, if the same substance can help you avoid cancer and diminish joint pain, then preventing everyday infections as a side effect is pretty convenient.

Along this line, and in the never ending quest to use curcumin to its fullest, it has even been incorporated into textiles. Combined with aloe vera, it is thought to act as a microbial suppressant in cotton, wool and rabbit hair fabrics. After 30 cycles through a home washing machine, curcumin wool still was able to inhibit *Staphylococcus Aureus* up to 45% and *E coli* up to 30%.[13]

So again, what is the take-home message?

"To conclude, the present research findings suggested that curcuminoids may act as an effective therapeutic candidate against age-associated mitochondrial impairment and thus may promisingly delay aging and associated neurodegenerative disorders."[14]

 SCORE!

Drawbacks

It is inevitable that our seemingly perfect hero has a flaw... and that flaw is bioavailability. Standard curcumin is lipid soluble, and much like several other lipid soluble agents, it does not get absorbed well into the body. As well, once there, it is rapidly metabolized and quickly eliminated. People just can't consume enough of the stuff to maximize its benefits. Standard curcumin blood levels peak at 2 hours, but are gone by 4.5 hours, giving it a half life of 2.6 hours.

However, because the potential for benefit is so high, researchers are working diligently, if not greedily, to develop the perfect form for oral intake.

In the first go around, it was packaged with pepper, or piperidine. This system worked by inhibiting the breakdown of the curcumin in the liver by blocking its glucuronidation. Studies around 1998 showed this significantly increased the bioavailability. In fact, 20 mg of piperidine with 2 gm of curcumin increased the bioavailability by 20-fold. The half life however, was still about 2.2 hours.

More modern attempts have incorporated it into nanoparticles, liposomes, micelles and phospholipid complexes.

Meriva is a phosphatidylcholine-curcumin complex that gets more readily incorporated into cell membranes. In a small study, 450 mg of Meriva was equivalent to 4 gm of standard curcumin; and in fact, the curcumin absorption was 29% higher.

Longvida is a form of curcumin developed at UCLA, using SLCP technology. Standing for "Solid Lipid Curcumin Particle" technology, it is touted to deliver higher levels of the product. Testing has in fact shown it to be 65 times more bioavailable than standard curcumin.

Biocurcumax or BCM 95 CG is yet another incarnation. Studies have shown it to be 6.93 or 7 fold more bioavailable than standard curcumin. As compared to regular curcumin, this formulation peaks at 2 hours, but is gone by 8 hours with a half life of 4.9 hours.[15]

Metacurcumin is a super curcumin made by a company called RevGenetics that packages the curcumin in a micelle, and has the highest absorption rate (277 X that of regular curcumin), fastest absorption rate and highest plasma concentration after 24 hours.

Safety?

• •

"The safety, tolerability, and non toxicity of curcumin at high doses are well established by human clinical trials."[9]

• •

Curcumin has the advantage of time in this category. It has been consumed for millennia. It is also considered to be "generally recognized as safe" by the FDA. Of the few side effects noted, huge quantities may result in diarrhea, a headache, a rash, or yellow stool.

Sounds like a small price to pay!

Kaufmann Number: 2.3.1.0.3.0.3

CHAPTER 15:

CARNOSINE

Magic.

If you take old and grumpy human cells that are near to retirement and put them in a bath of carnosine, they become young again.

If you give carnosine to aging mice, they remain youthful and live much longer. Chronologically old rats keep their shiny, sexy fur coats and they remain physically active and are quite virile.

If you give carnosine to athletes, their performance improves.

If you give carnosine to old humans, they are less depressed and more active.

If you put carnosine into the eyes of people with cataracts, their vision improves.

Skin improves, wound healing is accelerated, telomere damage is reduced...

Too good to be true?

"As it turns out, not only can we reverse the aging process at the cellular level now, and actually do it quite simply and QUICKLY - but we can also reverse aging at the systems level and the organ level. And for that matter, we can reverse it in terms of how we look and feel- and by that I mean our skin and hair and energy levels. And then, of course, we can even reverse aging in terms of lifespan."[1]

"What's the secret? I'm talking about L-carnosine."[1]

Other catchy quotes:

Carnosine can "maintain health, enhance physical exercise performance and PREVENT AGING."[2]

"Carnosine and its imidazole-containing dipeptide derivatives are renown for their anti-aging, antioxidant, membrane protective, metal ion chelating, buffering, anti-glycation/transglycating activities."[2]

Magic? Maybe. At least the scientific version of magic.

Carnosine in its simplest form is a dipeptide, made up of L-histidine and β-alanine. That's it. Two simple ingredients. It exists in the brain and muscle in people, and generally speaking, we have no idea what it is supposed to do.

Throughout the animal kingdom, it exists in a variety of forms and in hugely varying quantities. Slightly different compounds, called carnosine analogs as they are so closely related, are anserine and ophidian. Anserine was originally identified in goose and chicken muscle (thus the name... anserine = goose like). Ophidian was identified in snakes, while the identical molecule in whales was called balenine. These are all considered histidine-containing dipeptides or HCD's and are thought to be parallel in function. Interestingly, almost all mammals have at least two of these molecules in their muscles. The pig and the buffalo have all three. Humans, for whatever reason, have only one.

In the fish world, marlin and salmon are the winners in terms of absolute quantity, while cod and tilapia fall far behind.[3]

Of note, whales and wallabies have extremely high levels.

In humans, carnosine is found only in muscle and in the olfactory bulb (the area responsible for smell) in the brain. Only 1% is actually in the brain, which is another mystery. So essentially this stuff is either muscle bound or floating around in the plasma. The amount per human also varies to a huge degree, with a three to four fold difference between individuals.

Carnosine is usually manufactured in muscle, by the enzyme carnosine synthase, utilizing the amino acids alanine and histidine. These come from our diet, and usually from animal products. The highest amounts are found in chicken, turkey, and tuna while lesser concentrations are in beef, pork, deer and rabbit.

• •

The healing capability of chicken soup apparently is not a myth as the carnosine levels rise after its consumption. Human intake of chicken soup or other forms of chicken have actually been shown to decrease the formation and growth of influenza virus.[4]

• •

Vegetarians, generally not consuming enough amino acids, do not fare as well in the carnosine department, and require other sources of direct carnosine or its building blocks. In general, vegetarians have 20% or less carnosine in their bodies as compared to omnivores.[3]

So, what exactly do we know about carnosine?

A Russian scientist, V. S. Gulewitch identified the stuff in 1900 from a meat extract. That was over a hundred years ago, so you would think we would have a better understanding of its purpose after all this time. Alas, we don't. We have however, discovered some really cool things that it can do.

In 1994, a couple of Australian scientists (McFarland and Holliday)[5] did a really amazing experiment, which I'll outline here:

1. They took senescent, i.e., old, but still functioning, human fibroblast cells and put them into a bath of carnosine. Very quickly, the old cells exhibited a rejuvenated appearance. They didn't just look younger though, they acted younger. Geeks would say the scientists converted senescent cells back to juvenile phenotypes.

2. Interestingly, the effect was short lived because if the carnosine was removed, the cells became old again. Fortunately, if the carnosine was reintroduced, the transformation recurred.

3. The cells in carnosine lived longer as well, in fact almost 300% longer than regular cells.

4. Cells normally stop dividing after a certain number of replications. Carnosine cells meanwhile had a 25% increase in the ability to keep dividing.

This is truly magic.

Just makes you want to bathe yourself in this stuff!

Not content to believe in magic, scientists all over the world, but especially in Russia, have spent lifetimes trying to untangle the mystery of carnosine.

• •

It seems different cultures love certain adjuvants. The Japanese love astaxanthin. The Indians love curcumin. The Russians love carnosine.

• •

The next living model, beyond cells anyway, to be experimentally subjected to carnosine were mice; specifically mice that were genetically programmed to age faster than regular mice (SAM=senescence-accelerated mice). When the Russians added carnosine to their diet, it "...attenuated the development of senior features and increased the lifespan by 20%."[6]

Interestingly, these same mice had a significantly greater number of spermatogonia and Sertoli cells. Thus, the reproductive ability (or manliness) of these mice was increased as well.

In 2003, Dr. Marios Kyriazis wrote a book entitled "Carnosine and other elixirs of youth… The miraculous anti-aging supplement."[7] I'm not really sure if it caught on in popular culture, but this guy did a really good job of explaining what the stuff is and why it's so cool. Perhaps society wasn't ready to believe it, but they should have. Not only were his claims valid, but in the last ten years the information has only become

more supported and incredible.

So, what does carnosine do in muscle? Why do we have this stuff in the first place?

Despite the fact that we don't really know its purpose, the best guess is that it serves as a buffer in the muscles. Under the conditions of high intensity muscular contractions, anaerobic glycolysis leads to the production of lactic acid, which of course, is an acid. The resulting pH can dip down to 6.5 (7.0 being normal) and lead to dysfunction of the proteins. Muscle then becomes fatigued, and it eventually leads to that burn that you feel. Acting as a buffer, that is an acid sponge, carnosine can block this muscle failure and allow for better or more consistent functioning in times of stress.

In a very Frankenstein-ish experiment, Severin, another Russian scientist, amputated frog legs and attached them to nerve stimulators (he called this a nerve-muscle preparation to make it sound a little less bizarre). Stimulating the nerve causes the muscle to contract and the leg to move. Eventually, this activity slows down if you stimulate it too much, i.e., it exhibits muscle fatigue. If, however, you put the experiment in a carnosine bath, this "offsets the fatigue." Now called Severin's phenomenon, it was yet more proof that carnosine was magical or at least an incredibly effective muscle buffer.

In 1938, it was proposed that the dipeptide could account for up to 25% of the buffering capacity in working muscle, and 40% in resting muscle. Since then, we have determined that the amount of carnosine is highest in fast twitch or type II, white fibers versus the slow twitch type. This makes sense, the faster a muscle is expected to work, the faster it becomes acidic and thus the more buffer it requires.

In the real world, athletes that excel in sprint-type or high intensity, but quick exercises have a naturally greater quantity of carnosine. These are the sprinters and short-track skaters for example. Endurance athletes meanwhile have a lot less, but still more than regular couch potato folks. So, in general we say that in short term exercises, carnosine causes in a delay of the onset of fatigue in the neuromuscular system, and raises the aerobic threshold.[4]

There is also a big difference in who has how much carnosine. Men, for example, have between 22-82% more than women.

It's truly not fair!

Before puberty, the sexes are roughly equivalent, then the boys just get more. Bodybuilders have a ton, castrated male mice have a lot less. Interestingly, girl mice given testosterone increase their carnosine levels by 268%.

Age is also significant. The older we get, the less carnosine we have. There is, on average, a 63% decline between the age of 10 and 70. This of course is true for all things leading to aging; whatever seems to help us, diminishes with time.

All right, so carnosine is good for muscles, but clearly this effect has little to do with not aging. What exactly does it do?

• •

> "Due to its antioxidant, protective, chelating, anti-glycation activity, this dipeptide can be used to prevent and treat diseases such as diabetes, neurodegenerative diseases, diseases of the sense organs and cancers."[4]

> "Carnosine appears able to extend the lifespan of cultured cells, rejuvenate senescent cells, inhibit the toxic effects of amyloid peptide..., inhibit glycosylation of proteins and protein-DNA and protein-protein cross linking, and maintain cellular homeostasis."[8]

• •

Let's run the list:

DNA / Information Systems: Telomeric Stability

If you recall from the DNA section, telomeres are the end caps on chromosomes that have recently been associated with length of life. That is, the longer the telomeres, the longer you can expect to live. You will also recall that with every cell division, the telomeres get a bit shorter.

Carnosine has been shown to reduce the telomeric shortening rate in cultured human fibroblasts.[13] It doesn't exactly make them longer, but they didn't lose much length.

As of yet, there is no human evidence to support this, but I'm sure the Russians are working on it.

Mitochondria / Energy systems: Free radical scavenging

Back to the evil free radicals we addressed earlier. As you may be tired of hearing, free radicals are a side product of mitochondrial activity and are detrimental to our very existence. I'm not going to expound on this concept again, only to note that it is huge in the process of aging. Luckily, carnosine is a potent scavenger of both reactive oxygen and nitrogen.

Under physiological conditions, rats given carnosine were found to not only have reduced oxidative damage, but carnosine could also improve the rats own endogenous antioxidants. It improved both the enzymatic and non-enzymatic abilities of the rats; for example, it restored depleted levels of glutathione and increased the basal levels of superoxide dismutase.[9]

A lot of rat brains were sacrificed for that small sentence! ▶ By very complex measurements that I'm not going to go into, carnosine was found to significantly decrease oxidative stress in the brain.

• •

In fact, "Carnosine, the natural dipeptide B-alanine-L-histidine, meets almost all requirements for an ideal antioxidant."[10]

• •

Waste Management: AGE reduction

The other and probably most important quality of carnosine is its ability to block AGE formation (you may want to glance back at the Waste Management chapter). Recall that glycation is the nonenzymatic bonding of glucose to other molecules. After this first step, there are a series of other, more complex molecular rearrangements that ultimately lead to the nonreversible attachment of AGEs to collagen and other key structures. We have seen that this occurs all over the body, and is huge yet again in the aging process.

It turns out that carnosine blocks some of the intermediate steps of this process. This sounds like yet another drab geeky detail, but in reality, this is phenomenal. Even better, while study after study demonstrates the ability of carnosine to block the formation of AGE products, there is even some indication that the already damaged, cross-linked and thus decommissioned proteins can actually be rescued. So, there is limited, but strongly suggestive evidence, that we can in fact turn back the clock in terms of collagen damage. This is also key as there are very few substances that have this capability, and none that are over the counter and without side effects.

• •

"The ability of carnosine to prevent AGEs and ALEs formation is mediated by different mechanisms, and this is due to the fact that AGEs and ALEs formation is a quite complicated pathway, involving different reaction mechanisms and several catalyzing agents."[3]

"Carnosine was found to be effective already in the first step of AGE formation as well as by reversing glycated protein through a transglycation mechanism."[3]

"Carnosine can inhibit cross-linking of proteins and protects against the inactivation of enzymes induced by glycation, oxidation and a steroid."[11]

"In vivo studies using different animal models have clearly demonstrated the ability of histidine-dipeptides to inhibit AGEs formation and prevent RAGE activation."[12]

• •

Enough said by very smart scientists; you get the picture, but you need to realize that this is crucial. I said it above, and I'll say it again. There are very few substances that have this ability, therefore it is absolutely key in our anti-aging regime.

What body parts does this effect?

Of course carnosine is effective all over the body, but it's fun to examine some of the more impressive findings.

The Brain

Carnosine is thought as well to have a protectant effect on most neurons, both in and out of the brain. Interestingly, carnosine when given to rats,

Not a bad idea if you like loud rock concerts! ▶ protected them from loud, or acoustic trauma. Much like nicotinamide riboside, the nerve cells or nuclei of cochlear cells were preserved.[4]

Behavior is also a component of the brain, and it too can be influenced by carnosine. It is known to effect behavior in chickens and rodents, and is known to suppress anxiety in rats.[6]

In a bizarre experimental called "forced swimming," i.e. swim until you drown, rats that had been given carnosine were significantly less depressed than otherwise almost drowned rats.[15]

Human studies have actually demonstrated an enhancement of cognition as well as the feeling of well-being in several types of folks. Specifically it was beneficial for autistic children, Gulf War solders with PTSD, and it improved the signs and symptoms of schizophrenia.[14]

Eyes

Another really cool effect is in the eye. The lens of the eye is normally clear and sits just inside the pupil (we talked a bit about this in the chapter on astaxanthin). When the lens functions normally, it expands and contracts to focus the penetrating light on the retina at the back of the eye.

Over time, the proteins in the lens fail, the structure gets stiff and one develops presbyopia, or the inability to focus up close. The lens can also get hazy or opaque, and develops what are called cataracts. These issues arise as a consequence of the proteins, mostly α-crystallin, aggregating or cross-linking abnormally.

As of 2010, cataracts were the leading cause of blindness in the world. Risk factors (in case you are wondering about your own risk) include smoking, prolonged UV exposure, diabetes and a high body mass index. Essentially anything that increases oxidative stress or glycation stress can precipitate cataract formation.

The Russians, mesmerized by carnosine, discovered that there is a lot of the substance in youthful lenses.[17] Over time, of course, the quantity of carnosine diminishes.

In an astonishing discovery, it was determined that carnosine, if delivered or replenished in the lens, could inhibit the α-crystalin aggregation. This demonstrated that carnosine could block the formation of cataracts. Even more incredible, however, is that carnosine can actually disaggregate or reverse the glycation of the α-crystallin. I'll say it again…it can REVERSE it.

For the first time ever (plus the addition of astaxanthin), there is actually a way to improve your vision.

Getting the carnosine into the eyes was the next trick. Luckily, Russians are not only smart, but persistent. They discovered that a slightly modified form, N-acetyl carnosine (NAC), can be delivered via eye drops and that it actually gets into the lens.

At this point, innumerable studies (one with 50,500 people) with NAC drops have demonstrated improvement in visual acuity for people with cataracts, decreased glare sensitivity, and even color perception. They "promote vision health and prevent vision disability from senile cataracts, primary open-angle glaucoma, age-related macular degeneration, diabetic retinopathy, and aging."[18]

To sum it up, "NAC eye drop therapy is the crown jewel of the anti-aging medical movement and revolutionizes early detection, treatment, and rejuvenation of age-related eye-disabling disorders."[18]

• •

"Also, carnosine seems to delay the impairment of eyesight with aging, effectively preventing and treating senile cataract and other age-related diseases. Therefore, carnosine may be applied to human beings as a drug against aging."[8]

• •

Wound Healing

Improved wound healing is also a side feature of carnosine. The etiology remains unknown at this point, but hypotheses include either an increase in the building block amino acids, an increase in the fibroblastic growth factor, or even improved collagen stimulation. What is known however, is that supplementation with carnosine is extremely beneficial. Studies have shown that it doubles the rate of repair in injured guinea pig lung, and even in human lungs that are injured by treatment with bleomycin, a chemotherapy agent.[3]

Utilizing this wound healing ability, Japanese scientists have jumped on the bandwagon. Combining carnosine with zinc and naming it Z-103, they proved that it could accelerate the healing of stomach ulcers. As well, Japanese physicians are prescribing carnosine to radiation patients because it reduces the radiation damage to the skin.[10]

Skin

First, the ugly truths.[19]

"Collagen undergoes progressive browning with aging and diabetes, characterized by yellowing, fluorescence and cross linking."

"Browning reactions accumulate gradually with advancing age in long-lived tissue proteins."

"We now know that between 40% and 50% of skin aging is caused by glycation - the damage directly resulting from eating sugar. It's one of the worst skin agers; more than sun, more than the environment."[16]

Therefore, a three month supplementation study with carnosine was conducted, and its results impressive: " ...the skin parameters investigated showed a continuous and significant improvement as compared to the placebo."

"The finding that already-formed AGE cross-links can be pharmacologically severed and attendant pathology thereby reversed by non-hydrolyzed carnosine... has broad implications for the skin beautification....and skin diseases associated with aging."[19]

Ok, carnosine seems to be hugely beneficial, but can you actually increase the amount of carnosine in your body? Of course!

Studies have shown that you can increase your muscle content up to 80% after 10 to 12 weeks of supplementation. The levels also tend to remain elevated in the muscle once the supplementation has stopped. The washout period is also very slow, so once good levels of carnosine are reached in the muscle, they stay put for a while. The decline occurs at about 2-4% per week,[20] so it can last for up to 10 to 20 weeks.[3]

If you are looking for elevations in muscle carnosine only, then the supplementation with β-alanine by itself is fine. To increase the circulating levels of carnosine however, and thus enjoy the actual anti-aging effects, you must ingest carnosine in its entirety.

Things to be concerned with:

As adults, there is no indication that large doses of carnosine have any negative effect on the body. In children however, this is not the case.

There exists, in most of us, an enzyme that splits carnosine back into its pieces. Carnosinase actually comes in two forms, serum carnosinase and tissue carnosinase, and they are both located on chromosome 18. The presence of this enzyme matters for two reasons.

If a child is born without the enzyme (serum carnosinase deficiency), they develop carnosemia, meaning too much carnosine in the blood. This can lead to progressive mental retardation in children, which clearly is a bad thing.

The other reason this enzyme is important is that it controls the amount of carnosine we can keep circulating in our bodies as supplementing adults. We have to intake enough to overcome its breakdown. Interestingly, this does not effect the muscle storage of carnosine, because it doesn't matter if you intake supplemental carnosine or just alanine. The carnosinase breaks down the carnosine into histidine and alanine, the alanine gets taken up into the muscle and the level of carnosine rises regardless.

The side effects of carnosine supplementation are very low. Some people do however report a mild paresthesia, or prickly sensation in the skin mostly in the face and head, arms and hands. With large single doses, the tingling can start within 20 minutes or so, but it usually dissipates within the hour.

This effect can be reduced or avoided by taking less supplement more frequently.[20]

The other good news is that carnosine is not addictive, there is no danger of overdose, and it does not accumulate in the organism during long-term administration because its surplus is cleaved by the enzyme carnosinase.[10]

Where can you get carnosine? Pretty much anywhere. It is a rather inexpensive dipeptide that is available over the counter. Recommended doses are somewhere between 500 to 1000 mg per day. You can also get N-acetyl carnosine eyes drops over the counter, and stave off your failing vision.

Kaufmann Number: 0.3.0.0.0.0.3

CHAPTER 16:

METFORMIN

• •

"Common drug has the potential to slow aging, boost cancer recovery."[1]

"Metformin: Do we finally have an anti-aging drug?"[2]

• •

Clark Kent of the drug world, metformin is seemingly old fashioned and benign. It's been around forever; but underneath…special powers!

Metformin. It just sounds old. Old people consume it in monstrous quantities. In fact, there is a very high probability that your parents or grandparents are already on the medication as millions of older folks are. Associated with diabetes and consumed by the masses all over the world, the circumstances around this medication turn out to be quite fortuitous for the rest of us. Because so many people have been on the drug for so long, we have an excellent record from which to determine side effects, efficacy and especially the unexpected outcomes that now we can appreciate.

For example, a 2014 study retrospectively studied Type 2 diabetics on either metformin or sulfuronureas (a different type of glucose-controlling agent) and compared them with non-diabetics on neither of these drugs. In a study of 150,000 people, the type 2 diabetics on metformin had higher survivability. Let me rephrase…the diabetics did better than non-diabetics.[3]

In fact, among patients in their 70's, mortality was reduced by 15% in the metformin group. This seems preposterous; everyone knows that diabetes kills people. Between the heart attacks, strokes and generalized poor health, diabetes is bad. On the other hand, metformin was able to not only help these people, but they had BETTER survivability than non-diabetics (the folks on sulfuronureas didn't do so well by comparison). This study in fact sparked the interest of innumerable scientists who then set out to determine what metformin could do for non-diabetics.

But first, a little perspective.

The drug has been on the market since the 1950s, and is generally taken by the older, weight-challenged crowd; but, it turns out that our Clark Kent of a medication can improve lifespan, health span, reduce the risk of cancer, and help with weight loss… for all of us. And get this, the other important thing to note is that the side effect profile is minimal. Compared to most medications available today, there is very little to worry about.

So, lets take off Clark's glasses and examine him more closely.

$$\begin{array}{ccc} NH & NH \\ \| & \| \\ N{-}C{-}N{-}C{-}NH_2 \\ | & | \\ & H \end{array}$$

Metformin is a biguanide (N,N-Dimethylimidodicarbonimidic diamide), also known by the trade name Glucophage. Earlier use of the plant, *Galega officinalis* or the French Lilac, was documented in Medieval Europe as an herbal remedy for diabetic symptoms.

Metformin was officially discovered in 1922, but human studies didn't begin until the 1950s. It was then that the French physician Jean Sterne introduced it to her countrymen as a prescription medication in 1957. The compound debuted in the United States in 1995. Two similar but more potent compounds, phenoformin and buformin were available for a while, but were pulled from the market in the 1970s secondary to pretty terrible side effects.

At first, metformin was not a popular medication. Coming to the market at roughly the same time as insulin for the treatment of diabetes, insulin proved to be more widely utilized. This made clinical sense at the time because mimicking an endogenous substance like insulin should be far better than introducing a new, non-endogenous drug. Regardless, the medication finally caught on and it has been in use ever since. Because of this long history, we know that it is safe as a glucose lowering agent without the risk of the blood sugar becoming too low, i.e., hypoglycemia.

Over the course of time, metformin has evolved to become the first line therapy for Type II diabetes.

• •

Type I diabetes is an autoimmune disease, usually effecting younger people, that has nothing to do with being overweight or having metabolic syndrome. The body makes antibodies that attacks the pancreas such that insulin cannot be produced normally.

Type II diabetes is much more prevalent, and is associated with being overweight, aging and having a poor diet.

• •

As of 2015, there were 382 million people with diabetes globally, 85-95% of which were Type 2. Meanwhile, 150 million people were on metformin. So, when you consider which adjuvants to add to the anti-aging regime, know that the side effect profile of metformin has been well established. Rest assured here, millions of people have come before you.

The other thing you are probably asking about now is what does this have to do with me? I don't have diabetes, you say. I ask for patience, please.

So, what exactly does metformin do? It turns out, a lot of things.

• •

"The anti diabetic drugs.......and metformin were shown to reduce hyperglycemia, improve glucose utilization, reduce free fatty acid utilization, (reduce) gluconeogenesis, serum lipids, insulin, and IGF-1, reduce body weight and decrease immunodepression both in humans and rodents."[2]

• •

DNA / Information Systems

Metformin, determined to be an overachiever in every category, does several things for our DNA. First, it protects it from harm. It is not entirely clear how this works, but it is probably associated with the reduction in oxidative stress.

• •

"Results showed that metformin reduced age- and oxidative stress-related accumulation of DNA damage" in intestinal stem cells from *Drosophilia.*[4]

"The results of the present study validate the effectiveness of metformin, alone or with the addition of resveratrol, in reducing the risk of aging by conferring protection against UV-induced DNA damage."[5]

• •

Metformin also acts as an epigenetic modular; it induces genome-wide DNA methylation, but in a manner unlike the other agents. It modulates the activity of S-adenosylhomocystein hydrolase,[6] which is an enzyme in the methylation cycle.

Evidence also exists that metformin is able to promote DNA damage repair. The details, however, are a little lacking.

Lastly, there is a phenomenal, 2013 review article concerning metformin that lists several benefits to DNA. These include decreasing genomic instability, increasing DNA repair efficacy and even stimulating telomeric length. I haven't found corroborating evidence for the last one, but it would be fantastic if it were true.[2]

Mitochondria / Energy Systems

Metformin is well known to activate our own, endogenous antioxidants. This however, occurs through a pathway we have yet to discuss, the Nrf2-ARE, (nuclear factor-like 2 - Antioxidant Response Elements).[7] The details of this are not important, except to note that it has significant control over the endogenous antioxidants that we have come to know and love: heme-oxygenate-1, glutamate cysteine ligase, glutathione S-transferase, glutathione peroxidase, superoxide dismutase, catalase, sulfiredoxin and thioredoxin.

Pathways: Activates AMP Kinase

In 2001, it was established that metformin did far more than just lower blood sugar. It turns out that it stimulates AMP Kinase in liver cells. Realizing that this doesn't sound very exciting, it actually is.

AMP Kinase is a master regulator of cellular energy homeostasis that determines what the entire body does with its energy; but, alas, you already know all of this.

Let's back up a minute and review for a second anyway. In a nut shell, metformin gets transported into the liver or hepatic cells and accumulates in the mitochondrial matrix. Once there, it selectively inhibits complex I of the mitochondrial respiratory chain. If you recall, this chain is necessary for the production of ATP from AMP. The cell is able to detect the ratio of AMP (low energy state) to ATP (high energy). When the energy is low, as happens when the system gets a little blocked, the cells principle energy sensor, AMP Kinase gets activated.

All right, so metformin stimulates AMP Kinase. Then what?

Stimulating AMP Kinase puts cells on the pathway to mimic caloric restriction.

Again, in case you have forgotten, "CR has been shown to increase resistance to stress and toxicity, and to maintain youthful levels of function and vitality in laboratory mammals at advanced chronological age."[2]

As an added bonus to prove that metformin is working, it turns out that you can profile specific gene patterns that occur in various situations. And, as you have guessed, the gene profiles seen under conditions of caloric restriction match those triggered by the use of metformin.

Another of the benefits of activating AMP Kinase that were mentioned in a previous chapter but you may not remember, have to do with lipids and fat storage. Metformin has proven extremely beneficial in improving lipid metabolism.

Since the levels of glucose are lowered, lipids become a prime target as an energy source. Not only does the body utilize stored fat preferentially over glucose, metformin also prevents lipogenesis, the formation of new fat. Again, as a geeky aside, you can actually measure a reduction in the gene transcription of fatty acid synthase, a necessary enzyme to create new fats.[8]

Quality Control

There is some evidence that metformin increases the efficacy of DNA repair mechanisms.

Immune system/Security: Anti-inflammatory

Although not a major mode of operation, metformin also acts on the inflammatory pathway through several channels.

"Metformin blocks the activity of the transcription factor Nuclear Factor -$\kappa\beta$ (NF-$\kappa\beta$) resulting in decreased secretion of pro-inflammatory cytokinesis by senescent cells."[9] In a mouse study, NF-$\kappa\beta$ was in fact decreased by 64%.

Very recently, metformin was also found to decrease the inflammatory system by inhibiting the differentiation of monocytes to macrophages. You don't really need to know this, but the differentiation is a pivotal step in the early immune response. "In response to injury or inflammatory stimuli, migration of circulating monocytes into the inflamed tissue is accelerated, and subsequent differentiation into macrophages occurs rapidly."[10]

• •

> *"Conclusively, the anti-inflammatory benefits of metformin targeting macrophage differentiation/polarization may help explain its usage value for presentation and/or treatment of vascular injury, atherosclerosis, certain cancers, and insulin resistance."*[10]

• •

Individual Cell Health: Effects on stem cells

Despite the low turnover of neurons, we know that there is some turnover, especially in the hippocampus. Without this, not only would we all lose our minds much faster and sooner than we already do, but recovery from brain injury could never happen. Therefore, as a phenomenal bonus, we now know that metformin boosts the formation of new nerve cells.

• •

> *"Metformin, an FDA-approved diabetes drug, promotes proliferation, self-renewal, and differentiation of adult neural precursors."*[11]

> *"This finding has led to studies to repurpose metformin as a neurodegenerative agent to treat the injured or degenerating brain."*[11]

• •

Waste Management: Hypoglycemic effects (Lowering the blood glucose)

First and foremost, metformin lowers your blood glucose. Why is this a good thing?

We talked earlier about AGEs (in the Waste Management chapter) and the evils that they inflict upon the body. The first step in their production was the association of glucose with another molecule. So, it follows, we need to control the glucose.

Let's start with a quick review of glucose so we're all on the same page.

The body's main source of energy that gets distributed around the body is sugar, usually glucose or fructose. When the sugar reaches the individual cells, it gets converted into ATP. We can also run on energy from proteins and fats, but glucose is the preferred energy source. As such, the body has devised a very complex system of utilization, production, and storage of glucose that is tightly controlled. Most of this is guided by the liver, which senses the level of glucose available and directs the appropriate response.

At the beginning of its ingestion, glucose is absorbed from the gastrointestinal tract and travels around the body within the blood stream. The pancreas, sensing the glucose, produces insulin that is necessary as a cofactor to allow entry of glucose into individual cells.

Once glucose is circulating, some of it goes to use immediately. The liver extracts enough glucose to keep a 24 hour supply of energy and sensing any extra, it sends out signals to create fatty deposits in order to store the remainder. When the liver senses that the bodies levels are low, it takes energy out of storage and creates new glucose. This is called gluconeogenesis, that is the genesis of new glucose.

Generally speaking, the glucose control system is very tightly controlled and quite efficient. Over the course of millions of years where humanoids and other mammals rarely consumed enough calories or glucose, it was crucial to have tight metabolic control of energy supplies. In today's world, most of us consume far too many calories. The body responds with its ever efficient system, and soon fat tissue is stocked up in every available space. The pancreas also cranks out as much insulin as possible, trying to keep up with the challenge. Ultimately, the glucose intake overpowers the bodies ability to cope, and the amount of glucose in the blood rises.

On the absolute end of the high glucose spectrum, the high levels cause osmotic damage, cataracts, kidney damage, nerve damage, poor wound healing, blood vessel damage and innumerable other problems.

But even normal levels of glucose can cause damage over the course of decades. Even if the fat stores are within normal levels, there still is an abundance of glucose floating around in the blood stream. This glucose ends up bonding to whatever it touches. Like candy sticking to your teeth, the glucose adheres to lipids, proteins, structures, pretty much everything, essentially acting to caramelize the body from the inside out. These complexes, if you recall, are referred to as AGEs, Advanced Glycation End Products. The accumulation of these AGEs turn out to be a consistent biomarker of aging. And as could be predicted, the higher the blood glucose on a regular basis, the higher the production of AGEs.

Ok, so how exactly does metformin lower the blood sugar?

The first thing metformin does is reduce the amount of glucose that gets absorbed from the gut. Apparently metformin accumulates in the intestine at very high concentrations and thus has several effects here. It is not exactly clear how it occurs, but the intake from the GI tract gets reduced.

While we are in the gut, another interesting effect of metformin is that it "causes a profound shift in specific subsets of bacterial taxa."[9] Essentially, metformin alters the population of bacteria in your GI tract, selecting for bacteria that are more common in healthy, skinnier people. An increase in a bug called *Akkermansia municiphilia*, for example, improves the metabolic profile, reduces adipose tissue inflammation, and improves glucose control. *Lactobacilli* is also one of the bugs those populations increase with metformin. This bug utilizes the glucose itself, produces lactate which then gets taken to the liver. As a side note, this lactate is used by the liver to create new glucose thus preventing overt hypoglycemia.[9]

Thus, by altering the gut's resident bacterial population, the available glucose is reduced as well. This probably contributes to the decline in absorbed glucose.

Once metformin is absorbed, it accumulates in the liver where it suppresses gluconeogenesis. Thus, the body is unable to make new glucose and needs to find an alternative energy source.

Step one accomplished. Glucose levels are lowered.

How does this translate into organ systems? Here is but a sample of its diverse benefits.

Cardiovascular System

The most obvious and appreciated effects of metformin are on the cardiovascular system and especially metabolic syndrome. This is important to us for many reasons, but especially that "patients with metabolic syndrome exhibit many manifestations of accelerated aging."[7] Aging is bad enough, but accelerated aging is tragic!

Diabetes and the Metabolic syndrome combine to reduce lifespan secondary to the increased risk of heart disease, cardiovascular diseases, inflammatory diseases, and cancer among others. The good news is that metformin can prevent or delay the onset of all of these things, at least in mice,[7] as well as minimizing the secondary effects of diabetes. Therefore, our medication should be able to significantly improve health span, if not lifespan.

Following this line of thought, one of the most telling findings about metformin is that it can reduce cancer in diabetics. Diabetics have a significantly increased risk of breast, colon, prostate, kidney, and even pancreatic cancer,[8] so the issue is a big one. Luckily, metformin can help and not just a little, but a lot. Through the processes outlined above, diabetics on metformin have a 25 to 40% reduction in cancer. In fact, "Metformin already may have saved more people from cancer death than any drug in history."[2]

Pretty impressive! ▶ In human studies, metformin has already proven itself. In a retrospective trial in the UK, metformin therapy reduced the diabetes-related deaths by 42%, and the all-cause mortality by 36%.[8]

In a similar UK diabetic study, metformin lowered the risk of myocardial infarction (heart attack) by 39%.[9] As well, when a heart muscle died from an infarct, the degree of damage was reduced if the rat heart had been pretreated with metformin.

So, overall, metformin has proven to be superbly suited to treat and even prevent disease associated with cardiovascular diseases.

Menopause

Menopause is clearly a milestone in the lives of women, which some see as a blessing and some see as a curse. There is however, a direct correlation between the onset of menopause and age-related diseases such as atherosclerosis, osteoporosis and cancer. No one actually knows exactly why women go into menopause, but hypotheses abound. Regardless, in female mice, metformin was found to delay menopause.[13] Interestingly, caloric restriction has the same effect.

Another interesting disease that metformin seems to be useful for is polycystic ovary syndrome (PCOS). Effecting 5 to 15% of reproductive-aged women, it is associated with menstrual disturbances, hyperandrogenism and polycystic ovaries. Typically, these women have trouble getting pregnant. It turns out that metformin increases ovulation, improves menstrual cyclicity, and reduces the levels of serum androgens. How exactly metformin does this is still controversial.[8]

Skin

Not really relevant to aging, but perhaps falling into the category of better living, metformin has also been adopted by dermatologists to treat some rather unbecoming skin issues. These include (but are probably not limited to) hirsutism, acne, hidradenitis, acanthosis nigricans, eruptive xanthomas, psoriasis and even some skin cancers.[14]

Aging

Can it actually help us to stop aging?

Metformin can prolong the health span of worms, slows lipofuscin accumulation, extends mean lifespan and prolongs youthful locomotor ability in a dose-dependent manner.[2]

In mice, metformin tends to decelerate the age-related rise in blood glucose and triglyceride levels, it reduces the serum level of cholesterol and Beta-lipoproteins, delays menopause and extends the mean lifespan by 4 to 8%.[2]

The other thing we have learned from rodents is that the earlier the therapy is started, the better the outcome. Administration of metformin early in the lives of one set of rodents increased lifespan by 14%. Administration later in life had a reduced 6% effect. When initiated even later in life, it did nothing.

Whereas there presently are no studies confirming the ability of metformin to prolong life, there will be soon. Working on the assumption that one way to delay aging is to delay age-related diseases, Dr. Nir Barzilai, the Albert Einstein College of Medicine, and the American Federation for Aging Research (AFAR) are about to embark on a prospective study of metformin in non-diabetic elderly folks between 65 and 80 years of age to see if the normal diseases of aging can be postponed. Specifically they are looking at cancer, cardiovascular disease, diabetes, cognitive decline and of course, mortality. Called the TAME (Targeting Aging With Metformin) project, they plan on recruiting 3,000 volunteers and following them for 6 years. The expected cost of this extravaganza is estimated to be about 66 million dollars, so I suspect that everyone involved is expecting excellent results. Fingers crossed regardless (Unless you are reading this years later and the results are common knowledge).

In addition to determining if metformin can stand up to expectations, the study also is important in that it opens the door for medications to be approved to treat aging. Never before has aging been a disease, or something that needed to be fixed... until now.

What else do you need to know?

The dose of metformin in the quest of not aging is difficult to gauge. The treatment dose for diabetes falls somewhere between 500 to 2,000 mg per day.

Because this drug is a real medication, we know far more about it than most of the others. Thus:

- Oral bioavailability: 50-60%
- Peak plasma concentrations: 1 to 3 hours immediate release / 4-8 hours with extended-release formulations
- Uptake can be delayed 30 minutes if taken with food
- Protein binding in plasma: minimal
- Half life: 1.7 to 4.5 hours
- Excreted unchanged in the urine or through the GI tract

The drug blocks the metabolism of a few vitamins, so long-term therapy should be accompanied by the addition of supplemental B12 and folate. Sarcopenia can also be a byproduct of taking metformin. The addition of either branched-chain amino acids or leucine in particular can help to stave off this complication.

The side effects are generally not too bad. Most people get some sort of GI upset. Twenty-nine percent of people get transient diarrhea, abdominal pain, cramps and excess gas. Up to ten percent of folks abandon the therapy, but most people feel nothing and just live much better.

Of the actual, dangerous side effects, the most important is the possibility of lactic acidosis. The incidence is about 3 cases/100,000 patient years. Factors that increase this risk include age greater than 60, decreased liver, kidney or cardiac function, diabetic ketoacidosis, surgery, respiratory failure, ethanol intoxication and fasting. The good news is that anyone taking metformin as we are, that is just trying not to age, generally don't have these issues.

On a final note, sometime ago in the scientific literature a list evolved that is supposed to represent the 9 tentative hallmarks of aging mammals. These include:

Genomic instability, telomeric attrition, epigenetic alterations, loss of proteostasis, deregulated nutrient sensing, mitochondrial dysfunction, cellular senescence, stem cell exhaustion, and altered cell-to-cell communication.

As a last vote of confidence… "Metformin seems to influence them all."[2]

Kaufmann Number: 3.1.3.2.2.2.3

CHAPTER 17:

ALPHA LIPOIC ACID

Alpha Lipoic Acid is stealthy. It has never made the front page. Its name isn't catchy; in fact it's the opposite: "Lipo" means "related to fat," and "acid" sounds painful. Neither of these words sound inviting; and the combination makes it even worse. But alas, Alpha LA gets a lot done…stealthily. It's effective, but with very little fanfare or pizzazz.

Alpha Lipoic Acid goes by various names, none of which are very memorable. In this instance the names include thioctic acid, acetate replacing factor, billet, lipoicin, or pyruvate oxidation factor. Scientifically, it is 1,2 - dithiolane-3-pentanoic acid.

As such, I have come to believe that Alpha LA is a secret agent. She has no real name, no exceptional background story, she's just doing her job under the radar. She's not British, however, so she isn't a 00. She is simply Alpha… Alpha LA.

In the human body, Alpha LA resides mostly in the mitochondria, where very small quantities are produced endogenously from octanoic acid. Most of our Alpha LA, however comes from dietary sources. The substance is produced in the mitochondria of both plants and animals, with the majority coming from red meat, liver, heart and kidneys. In the plant world, spinach, broccoli and tomatoes yield the most, although there is significantly less than in the animal products.

 If you're a vegetarian, take note!

Because of its molecular arrangement, there are two possible isomers, R-Lipoic Acid and S-Lipoic Acid. In nature, only the R is active. When produced synthetically, however, both isomers are created, but only the R will be beneficial.

Alpha LA had a very inauspicious beginning.

As most agents do

It was first identified in the 1930s in potatoes as a necessary growth factor for specific bacteria; thus it was named the potato growth factor.

Not very sexy

In 1951 it was isolated from cow liver.

Even less sexy

It wasn't until the 1980s that its antioxidant properties were discovered. Since then, the list of its cellular attributes has flourished; yet it remains pretty low key.

There is even a rumor that Alpha LA can be used for treating toxicities from poison mushrooms and radiation contamination. Some claim it was used as a treatment after the Chernobyl disaster.

 But yet we'll never know

So, why is Alpha LA so special?

• •

> *"It is well-defined as a therapy for preventing diabetic polyneuropathies, and scavenges free radicals,...and restores intracellular glutathione levels which otherwise decline with age."[1]*

> *"LA has been described as a potent biological antioxidant, a detoxification agent, and a diabetes medicine; it has also been used to improve age-associated cardiovascular, cognitive, and neuromuscular deficits, and has been implicated as a modulator of various inflammatory signaling pathways."[1]*

• •

So, I believe it's time to publicly recognize all that Alpha LA can do for us. In other words we are going to bring our spy in from the cold.

DNA / Information systems: Epigenetics

As we have discussed, DNA suffers over time and in some ways has become our natural, ticking clock. There is some evidence that Alpha LA acts as an epigenetic modifier; specifically, it inhibits histone deacetylase.

• •

"LA supplementation inhibits histone deacetylase protein activity in vitro in rat astrocytes."[2]

• •

Secondly we need to address our telomeres. These, of course, are getting shorter with time and are proportional to our lifespan. There are a few substances that are known to be beneficial in this arena that activate our own endogenous telomerase (and will be discussed shortly). Alpha LA achieves the same outcome, but the mechanism of action is a little **It's a bit more stealthy** ▶ different.

In a watered-down nut shell, Alpha LA induces PCG-1α which then induces TERT, which in turn increases telomere length.

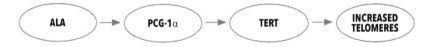

ALA ➝ PCG-1α ➝ TERT ➝ INCREASED TELOMERES

PCG= Peroxisome proliferator-activated receptor gamma coactivator-1α
TERT= Telomerase reverse transcriptase

• •

In cell cultures and in mice, "ALA treatment exhibited a prolonged stimulatory effect on telomerase activity, which is consistent with augmented TERT expression."[3]

"Ectopic expression of PGC coactivates TERT transcription, and reverses telomere malfunction and DNA damage."[3]

"Alpha Lipoic Acid stimulated expression of PGC-1α and TERT and reversed DNA damage, vascular senescence, and atherosclerosis."[4]

"Ectopic expression of TERT in adult and old mice increases health span and life span without increasing cancer incidence."[3]

• •

In an obese rodent study, the animals were shown to have reduced PGC and TERT expression, reduced telomerase activity, reduced SIRT1 and an increase in DNA damage. Remarkably, ALA supplementation prevented such reductions.[3]

Mitochondria/Energy systems: Antioxidant

Some have called Alpha LA the "Universal Antioxidant," others the antioxidant of antioxidants.[5] The substance is unique in that it is both water and fat soluble. Therefore, it has the ability to travel throughout the cell, including the membranes and the cytosol. Most of the other antioxidants are either one or the other, and thus have much less flexibility. This property also grants it access into the brain or nervous system, easily passing through the blood brain barrier.

In this category, Alpha LA helps out in three different ways. First, it serves both as a direct and indirect antioxidant. It is a free radical scavenger unto itself; and it also acts through the Nrf2 mediated system to activate the endogenous antioxidant enzymes.

In addition to this, Alpha LA has a unique ability; it intervenes and recycles used or "reduced" antioxidants. Thus, molecules such as Vitamin C, Vitamin E and glutathione can be used over and over in its presence.

• •

"LA is one such inducer of Nrf-2-mediated antioxidant gene expression and by so doing is able to significantly increase the cellular capacity of GSH synthesis."[6]

"Age related decreases in tissue GSH and/or reduced GSH/GSSH

(oxidized glutathione) ratios occur in different tissues such as brain, heart, and liver. LA reversed these age related changes and significantly boosted antioxidant systems."[6]

"Lipoic acid is a critical component of the antioxidant network because of its ability to regenerate other antioxidants, such as vitamin E and C, increase intracellular GSH levels, and provide redox regulation of proteins and transcription factors."[7]

• •

The traditional role of Alpha Lipoic acid is in energy production, acting within the mitochondria. It is a necessary cofactor for several reactions; without which there would be no energy production.

Specifically, Alpha LA is critical for the following, all essential for glycolysis or the TCA cycle.

• Pyruvate dehydrogenase
• A-keto-glutarate dehydrogenase
• Conversion of pyruvate to acetyl-CoA.

As you are already acutely aware, mitochondrial enzyme function declines with age. While this decline is multifactorial, the addition of supplemental Alpha LA can reverse many of the changes.

• •

"Aged rats given LA supplements showed a decrease in lipid peroxidation and an increase in the activities of mitochondrial enzymes, such as isocitrate dehydrogenase, a-ketoglutarate dehydrogenase, succinate dehydrogenase, NADPH dehydrogenase and cytochrome C oxidase. Moreover, no significant changes in mitochondrial enzyme activity were found in young rats treated with LA."[5]

"LA reverses the age-associated decline in mitochondrial enzymes."[5]

"Lipoic acid rescues the decline in mitochondrial bioenergetics associated with age."[8]

"Treatment with LA improved cognitive function through increased mitochondrial function in dogs."⁵

• •

Pathways: AMP Kinase Activity

The activity of Alpha LA on the AMP Kinase pathway is not straightforward. In fact, the effects differ depending on whether it is acting on peripheral tissues, or in the hippocampus.

In peripheral tissues, Alpha LA demonstrates the more classic behavior in that it activates AMP Kinase, and leads to increases in the sirtuin family, increases in NAD levels, etc. This is similar to the actions of metformin.

• •

"Lipoic acid was reported to increase energy metabolism and mitochondrial biogenesis in the skeletal muscle of aged mice by increasing the phosphorylation of AMPK."⁷

• •

Generally, as we are all aware, it is beneficial to activate AMP Kinase. However, Alpha LA does the exact opposite in the hypothalamus. In this setting, it actually suppresses AMP Kinase activity. The result of this however, is quite curious. It actually suppresses appetite. Therefore, Alpha LA is actually a reasonably potent appetite suppressant.

• •

"ALA exerts anorexic, anti-obesity effects by suppressing hypothalamic AMPK activity."⁶

• •

Immune system / Security: Anti-inflammatory

As we have discussed many times over, chronic inflammation is synonymous with aging. Therefore, anything that can stave off the inflammatory pathway is beneficial.

In this category, LA is a known inhibitor of Nuclear Factor-κβ.

• •

"LA inhibits NF-κβ activation independent of its antioxidant function."[6]

• •

If you recall, NF-κβ sits at the top of the inflammatory tree; thus Alpha LA should block the cascade as well. In fact, this holds true in the laboratory. Studies have demonstrated that LA decreases VCAM (vascular cell adhesion molecule), ICAM (intercellular adhesion molecule-1), as well as IL-6. It most likely decreases other inflammatory mediators as well, but no one has yet looked.

In asthma, or at least mouse asthma, dietary Alpha LA was able to reduce the hyper-responsiveness of the bronchial tree caused by inflammation. As well, it decreased the accumulation of inflammatory cells, i.e., eosinophils within the airway.[1]

Individual Cell Health

There is good evidence that hepatic and nerve cells in particular benefit from the presence of Lipoic acid. There is more about this below.

Waste Management: Insulin Mimetic

As we discussed in the waste management chapter, excess glucose in the body is detrimental. If you recall, it precipitates AGEs, which bind to and destroy proteins, lipids and DNA. The AGE complex then compromises the structural integrity of organs, as well as inciting system wide inflammatory processes. Therefore, anything that can

Under most circumstances ▶ lower blood glucose levels is beneficial.

Through a complex mechanism that is not entirely understood, Alpha

LA decreases blood glucose levels.

In cultured cells, our agent required one hour to induce its maximal effect on glucose uptake, which insulin can do in half the time. The delay suggests that it acts through secondary, presently unknown mediators. The effect is also not as potent as insulin and therefore should not lead to hypoglycemia; it does however help with the clinical control of diabetes.

• •

> *"Extensive evidence suggests that lipoid acid has potential therapeutic value in lowering glucose levels in diabetic conditions and that the intracellular redox status plays a role in the modulation of insulin action."*[7]

• •

Waste Management: Possible glycation blocker

The evidence here is a little thin. However, a few studies have shown that Alpha LA can block the glycation of albumin, i.e., sugar sticking to a serum protein. The agent was unable to protect low density lipoproteins however.[6] Regardless, this could prove very beneficial if it protected other molecules as well.

In general, our agent has demonstrated a wide skill set that can fend off the aging process. The effects should be body wide, but certain of the systems have taken precedence in the scientific literature.

Brain

Based on the ability of Alpha LA to cross the blood brain barrier, it was hypothesized that supplementation could protect the brain from the ravages of time, and so it has. LA has demonstrated a clear ability to improve learning and short term memory in aged rodents.[1]

• •

> *"LA can compensate for age-related, long term memory deficits in old rats and improve memory and learning in prematurely aged mice."[2]*

• •

Eyes

As an extension of the brain, the retina and optic nerve are particularly susceptible to photochemical and oxidative stress. Thus, there is well documented retinal and optic nerve degeneration over time. In a study beginning with already aged mice, (the ripe old age of 24 months), they were given Alpha LA and superoxide dismutase for 8 weeks. This combination was able to "counteract senile neurodegenerative deterioration to the retina and optic nerve."[9] There was increased stability in the mitochondrial membranes and less degenerative changes in the optic nerve as well.

This is truly impressive as damage to the eye structures is cumulative; it doesn't just start when we get old. Therefore, if we started protecting these structures prior to being old, we should theoretically be able to avoid the damage in the first place.

Bone

Osteoporosis is an imbalance between bone destruction from osteoclasts and bone rebuilding by osteoblasts. Whereas osteoporosis can afflict anyone, it is especially harsh on post menopausal women. Therefore, to model this situation, the ovaries were surgically removed from rats to create an estrogen deficiency situation. Under this circumstance, the rats developed osteoporosis. The supplementation with Alpha LA then was shown to increase bone density. As well, and as expected, it decreased the system wide, inflammatory markers TNF-α and IL-6. Alpha LA also decreased levels of osteopontin, a protein related to bone reabsorption.

In another study of rats fed high fat diets, Alpha LA supplementation resulted in increased bone mineral density, and an increase in the markers of increased bone formation, osteocalcin, as well as a decrease in gene transcription related to bone resorption activity.[10]

Liver

The effects of our agent were examined in rat livers, looking at actual microscopic structures and comparing young to old rats (4 months vs 24 months). From a tissue perspective, old livers were structurally demolished. They demonstrated sinusoidal collapse, endothelial thickening, blood congestion and other not so great changes. On a cellular level, old liver cells were hypertrophic, had cytoplasmic vacuoles (holes), had alterations in the organelles, and were crowded with lipofuscin. Of note, these changes were significantly ameliorated by Alpha LA supplementation.[11]

Diseases/Diabetes

The most studied disease that is currently being treated with LA is diabetes. In fact, LA has been a standard, prescribed medication for this disease for over 50 years in Germany.

This phenomena has been looked at extensively, with several well named trials. My favorites are the ALADIN study (Alpha-Lipoic Acid in Diabetic Neuropathy) and the SYDNEY trial (Symptoms of Diabetic polyneuropathy).

The outcomes demonstrate that between a combination of oral and intravenous Alpha LA, there was a significant improvement in feet and lower limb neuropathies (nerve dysfunction with numbness and burning).

As well, Alpha LA was shown to reduce blood glucose (which we knew), reduce high blood pressure and improve blood flow. It also improved the functionality of the nerves.

• •

"In animal models of diabetes, LA supplementation was reported to improve neural blood flow and nerve conduction."[5]

*"Alpha-lipoic acid has been shown to improve motor nerve
conduction velocity in experimental diabetic neuropathy and
protect peripheral nerves from ischemia in rats."[12]*

• •

Thus, it seems that Alpha Lipoid Acid would be a beneficial addition to our anti-aging regime. The question, then, is how much to take and what to be concerned with.

Presently, studies have pushed the consumed quantities higher and higher. At the moment, doses of up to 2,400 mg/day have had no adverse effects. As well, IV doses of 600 mg/day for 3 weeks have been equally benign.

High doses in rats can lead to sedation, including issues with apathy, eye closure and a hunched over posture.

Presently, supplements range from 200 to 600 mg daily, but there is no recommended dose.

The one thing to note however, is that unlike most of our supplements, LA should not be taken with food. It needs to be either a half hour before or two hours after in order to maximize its effects.

Kaufmann Number: **2.3.1.0.2.2.1**

CHAPTER 18:

APIGENIN

Apigenin is another of these substances that has been with humanity for thousands of years, but cleverly disguised as a tea. Despite that, it is also found in many herbs, including parsley, celery, onions, oregano and thyme.

Almost sounds like a Simon and Garfunkel song

The most consumed source, hands down however, is chamomile tea.

Prepared from the dried flowers from *Matricaria chamomilla*, chamomile tea deserves a few minutes of our time. It is also a cute, daisy-like flower.

Chamomile was first appreciated by the Egyptians, so much so that it was dedicated to the sun god, Rah. It was known, among other things, to increase healing rates and treat high fevers. Hieroglyphic records also show that chamomile was used cosmetically by Egyptian noblewomen, who applied crushed petals to their skin. The oil of chamomile was additionally utilized in the process of mummification.

This may be the very first time it was used in the quest for immortality... Although perhaps a little too late

The Greeks then adopted the plant. In fact, the name comes from this era as Chamomaela, and means "ground apple." Pliny the Elder mentions the similarity of the smell of the chamomile flower to the apple blossom, and this may be why the ancients used the term.

Not to be outdone, the Romans used chamomile to flavor drinks, treat wounds and make things in general just smell better.

The norsemen used it as a shampoo; apparently it made their braids shiny.

In the middle ages, chamomile became even more utilitarian. Medieval monks, for instance, suggested that people lie down on beds of chamomile flowers to reduce their depression. The flower petals were strewn about at gatherings to create pleasant odors. Chamomile was also used to flavor beer prior to hops.

Today, there are two types of chamomile, the Roman and the German. Roman chamomile, however, was not actually cultivated by the Romans, but was discovered growing wild by an English botanist in the Coliseum. He brought it back to England where it is one of the primary forms of chamomile now cultivated.

The German variety, meanwhile, is native to Europe and northwest Asia, where it still grows wild in addition to being cultivated. It is a bit different biochemically, and tends to be more medicinal than the Roman variety.

Traditionally, chamomile has been used for centuries as an anti-inflammatory, an antioxidant, a mild astringent and to heal wounds. Reviewing the list, it seems like chamomile was used to treat pretty much everything. On the other hand, there weren't that many choices way back when in Europe.

A brief list includes the following: wounds, ulcers, eczema, gout, skin irritations, bruises, burns, canker sores, neuralgia, sciatica, rheumatic pain, hemorrhoids, gastrointestinal disturbances including flatulence, indigestion, diarrhea, anorexia, motion sickness, nausea, and vomiting.

Externally, chamomile has been used to treat diaper rash, cracked nipples, chicken pox, ear infections, poison ivy, and disorders of the eyes including blocked tear ducts and conjunctivitis.

The tea is also supposed to be relaxing.

According to a popular website, "Chamomile eases the tension of excessive ego-desire... and the frustration, resentment and depression that frequently follow. It helps us to let go of fixed expectations, calmly acknowledge our own limitations, and more readily accept the help and support that others can manage to give us."

It's basically therapy in a cup!

Apparently the tea is also good for your life as a whole…

- Drinking chamomile tea is thought to instill positive energy and to bring prophetic dreams

- Burning chamomile each day is thought to bring you wealth

- Washing your hands with chamomile tea before gambling is thought to bring luck and success in your gambling endeavors

- Sprinkling chamomile over the thresholds of windows and doors is thought to repel negative energy or spirits

Peter Rabbit's mother even approved of the tea. After escaping Mr. McGregor's garden, she sends the mischievous young bunny to bed, with a cup of chamomile tea.

So, what exactly is chamomile tea?

The major chemical compounds include apigenin and alpha-bisabolol. However, there are approximately 120 secondary metabolites, including 28 terpenoids and 36 flavonoids. Of note, it also contains quercetin, (which is also on our list) and coumarins (which are not).

Thus, despite the fact that apigenin is one of the main active substances in chamomile, it certainly can't claim credit to all of the chemical effects.

Apigenin was also isolated from the tea in 1914, but has remained curiously under the radar ever since.

• •

Of note, if you don't enjoy chamomile tea, apigenin is in red wine and beer as well.

• •

What is apigenin?

Pretty simple
right?
Well, for starters its chemical name is 4', 5, 7,-trihydroxyflavone.

It is a flavone that exerts a "broad spectrum of activities, including DNA damage prevention, cell cycle arrest, and apoptosis induction, as well as immunomodulatory and anti-inflammatory effects."[1]

Let's run the list:

DNA / Information Systems: Epigenetic modifier

Again, I profess before any conversation about epigenetics, that it is easy to demonstrate molecular alterations and processes; it is much harder, however, to actually connect them with tangible results.

With that said, apigenin joins a special subset of adjuvants, the epigenetic diet, that are thought to turn back the epigenetic clock of sorts.

Very specific,
not quite sure
what it really
means in
the long run,
but at least
it sounds
scientific!
As such, apigenin reduces the expression or inhibits DNMT1 (DNA methyl transferases), DNMT3a, and DNMT3b.

Apigenin also inhibits some histone deacetylases in epidermal skin cells. This of course was discovered in a model of skin cancer, and the result of such activity was an up regulation of the Nrf2 signal pathway.[1]

As well, apigenin has been reported to inhibit histone deacetylases 1 and 3 in human prostate cancer cells. This resulted in a global histone H3 and H4 acetylation as well as localized hyperacetylation of histone H3.

Mitochondria / Energy Systems: Increases NAD

The only supplement that I am aware of that can do this, apigenin actually prevents the breakdown of NAD. As we learned in a previous chapter, NAD is an extremely important agent that is involved in innumerable cellular activities. It is involved in everything from DNA repair, to acting as a cofactor to the sirtuin family, to mitochondrial informational exchange. We also demonstrated that the supplementation of NAD could be extraordinarily beneficial. Therefore, the idea of having more NAD seems like a positive effect.

How does this occur? Apigenin inhibits CD38, a known NADase. Thus, blocking this enzyme blocks the breakdown of NAD, resulting in higher levels in the cells.[2]

• •

> *"Apigenin administration to obese mice increases NAD levels, decreases global protein acetylation, and improves several aspects of glucose and lipid homeostasis."[2]*

• •

Although the experts have decided this is beneficial, I feel I must voice a little bit of concern here. At the moment, it is not clear which cellular pathway is compromised by not utilizing the NAD. Clearly, NAD is required by all of the functions we have discussed. Thus, it is possible that some essential activity is being sub-optimized by this action.

On the other hand, as I said before, there is no harm in a few cups of tea.

Quality Control: DNA Repair

The evidence for this is a little thin. Even so, very few agents can assist in this category, so it could be a valuable attribute.

Apparently, "Apigenin can stimulate nucleotide excision repair genes to protect skin keratinocytes against UVB-induced skin inflammation."[3]

Immune Systems / Security: Anti-inflammatory

This category is much more precise. There is no doubt that apigenin can modulate the inflammatory pathway. As mentioned above, it activates the Nrf2 pathway.

• •

> *"Apigenin has been demonstrated to possess distinct anti-inflammatory activity in chronic inflammation and skin inflammation."[4]*

• •

Specifically, it modulates NF-κβ. If you recall, this sits at the top of our inflammatory tree. Thus blocking this cytokine essentially blocks almost the entire tree.

• •

> *"Apigenin inhibits the production of pro-inflammatory mediators such as IL-6, TNF-α, and IL-8 in several cell lines through NF-κβ signaling pathway."*[5]
>
> Apigenin is *"Thought to act through NF-κβ, inhibits pro-inflammatory mediators such as Prostaglandins, COX-2 and TNF-α."*[6]

• •

So, what interesting tricks can apigenin do?

There is always a cool trick. In this case, we find it in the skin.

As a brief review, skin is composed of mostly Type I collagen, in fact 80-85%. Type III collagen makes up between 10-15%.

Skin aging is associated with a disturbance in this collagen composition and metabolism. In general and for simplification, there is decreased production of collagen.

In a mouse model of skin aging, apigenin was injected in the skin. After one month, the dermal thickness and collagen density had significantly improved. Most importantly, there was an increase in both the collagen I and III.[3]

As well, the mice no longer needed selfie filters to look younger! ▶

Rather then injection, the topical treatment of apigenin in a different study, improved epidermal function by stimulating epidermal differentiation, lipid synthesis and secretion, as well as cutaneous antimicrobial peptide production.[3]

In one of the few human studies, Korean women over the age of 45 used apigenin cream daily for one month. The density of their skin improved, as did the elasticity, moisture, and evenness of the skin texture.[7] Clearly, the ancient Egyptian women knew what they were doing.

Of note, the Egyptians were also right about wound healing. Apigenin has been found to improve wound healing and tissue repair, at least in diabetic rats.

So, it appears that apigenin has earned a rightful position in our anti-aging protocol. How much to take? Again, hard to say, but adjuvants usually come in 20 to 50 mg capsules.

The only side effect of taking too much appears to be sleepiness. Thus, the FDA has categorized it as GRAS (generally recognized as safe).

Kaufmann Number: 2.1.0.1.2.0.0

CHAPTER 19:

SULFORAPHANE

The story of sulforaphane is a fascinating one. It is a story of discovery, hopefulness, creative packaging, and perhaps even, greed.

But let's start at the beginning. Once upon a time, not so very long ago, in fact in the 1990s, a great university announced that eating good foods was beneficial. Sounds a little ridiculous now, but in 1992 this was earth shattering.

Dr. Tony Talalay, at the Laboratory for Molecular Pharmacology at the John Hopkins University School of Medicine, discovered the health-promoting properties of a substance called sulforaphane glucosinolate in the *Brassica* family of vegetables, most notably, broccoli. What did this amazing substance do? Prevent cancer!

In 1992, these results were announced to the world. It made the front page of the New York Times and was listed as one of the top 100 discoveries of the 20th century by Popular Mechanics.

The study was, of course, done on rats, who after consuming broccoli sprout extracts for 5 days and then exposed to carcinogens, got less cancer than expected. Today, this is a bit less than front page news (Many, if not most, of all of the substances in this book might do the same). Remember, though, 1992 was a long time ago!

Since then, Dr. Tally did what any one of us would have done. He took his discoveries and went into private enterprise. He formed a company called Brassica Products, which now produces and sells specialized versions of his broccoli. Johns Hopkins, of course, receives a licensing fee from the company for each batch sold.

Clearly the folks at Hopkins aren't stupid!

Did he really discover the answer to cancer? Who knows, but since that time, thousands of studies on sulforaphane have been done, with very encouraging results.

Let's back up a bit first and talk about sulforaphane. It is an isothiocyanate, a molecule found in cruciferous vegetables, especially in broccoli, but it is also in kale, cabbage, and brussel sprouts.

I say that it is found in these veggies…but that is only partly true.

The components of this amazing substance are found in the vegetables, but they are contained in separate compartments. It turns out that sulforaphane is a rather unstable molecule; therefore, the plant keeps the two necessary components isolated until they are needed for whatever reason.

The first component is glucoraphanin, the biologically inactive precursor. This is housed apart, but within the same plant as its enzyme, myrosinase. When the plant cell ruptures, by some sort of trauma to the plant, (i.e., human chewing), the two mix and produce sulforaphane.

Why did this system develop? I have no idea. Clearly, it was evolutionarily important to either the plant or its natural ingestor. I'm sure some underpaid, biology grad student is trying to figure that out right now.

If you are said grad student, please call me! I'd love to know!

At the moment, however, it remains a mystery. It has however, initiated an arms race in the private sector to determine who might create the best and most stable formulation for to the public. Who won? Patience please…all in good time.

So, what makes this agent so special in the first place?

Presently, it is advertised to help fight cancer, autism, muscular dystrophy, asthma, and arthritis.

• •

>*"This compound protects against the onset or reduces the severity of cancer, retinal disease, and skin damage resulting from exogenous agents or genetic predisposition."*[1]

• •

It's that time again... to the list!

DNA / Information Systems: Epigenetic modulator

Whereas the idea of epigenetic modulation and the technology to investigate it didn't exist in the early 1990s, it was the prevention of cancer that initiated all the hoopla in the first place. Thus, for our purposes, let's assume this to be so (plus, I have frequently said I am not an oncologist and will not be offering any advice on cancer or its treatment).

However, we do know that sulforaphane does the following:[2]

1. Inhibits histone deacetylase, thus enhancing global histone acetylation.

2. Inhibits DNA methytransferases

3. Regulates micro RNA's (Micro RNA's are a bit complicated and I skipped over the explanation in the DNA section. I'm certainly not going to explain it here, but be aware that someday this may be important and thus I have included it as a basic fact.)

We know therefore, that our agent does indeed modulate epigenetics, and thus is included in our epigenetic diet.

Mitochondria / Energy systems: Antioxidant

There is little to no evidence that sulforaphane is a direct free radical scavenger. It does however, upregulate the endogenous antioxidants through Nrf2.

As well, "many animal studies show a significant decline in Nrf2 activity between youth and old age."[4] Again, no shocker here; anything that seems to be good for us, recedes over time.

• •

> *"Furthermore, its activity declines with age whilst up regulation of its activity by Nrf2 induction is describes as an avenue for maintaining cellular defenses with advancing age."[4]*

• •

How does sulforaphane stack up against some of our other NRF2 activators? According to the experts:

"Compared with widely used phytochemical-based supplements like curcumin, silymarin, and resveratrol, sulforaphane more potently activates Nrf2 to induce the expression of a battery of cytoprotective genes."[4]

There it is: Sulforaphane wins!

Quality Control: Organelle modulation and Autophagy

The in's and out's of this category are not clearly understood, but we do know that mitochondrial manipulation is crucial for cell survival. We know that the capacity to reorganize these and other organelles can increase the survivorship of the cell, and thus can help us as organisms. So what does sulforaphane actually do for the mitochondria? It modulates the number of functioning organelles.

The mitochondrial network and net energy production is determined by a regulated balance between fission and fusion. Fission is splitting of the mitochondria. When you need more energy, the cells simply divides one mitochondria, making two. On the other hand, if the mitochondria is defective or even is just no longer needed, it is either fused to another mitochondria, or selectively degraded by autophagy. The process of fusion allows for the sharing or recycling of cell resources.

• •

"In addition to stabilizing and activating Nrf2, SFN modulates mitochondrial dynamics and preserves cellular fitness and survival."[5]

• •

Individual Cell Health: Stem cell protection

The studies in this category are few and far between. Apparently, all of the scientists jumped on the cure cancer and decrease oxidation bandwagon. Thus, the stem cell activities were a bit ignored.

There are, however, a few good suggestive studies.

In one of these, mesenchymal stem cells were incubated with sulforaphane, at low doses that might be equivalent or achievable with an oral adjuvant. They discovered that these stem cells did much better. The sulforaphane promoted stem cell proliferation and protected the cells from apoptosis and senescence.[1]

There was a caveat however, excessive levels could have cytotoxic effects.

Thus far, sulforaphane has proven itself to be useful in the defense system against some cancers, and perhaps aging. The problem, of course, lies in the issue about the instability of the agent. Thus, there are endless blogs about how best to prepare broccoli in order to derive the greatest benefit.

One site says you must eat it raw and chew well. Another recommends heating to a certain temperature for only a few minutes; too long and the biochemicals are destroyed...too short and they aren't released. On top of this, if you destroy the enzyme myrosinase, all appears to be lost.

Note: not by me! ▶ Recommendations abound:

- First cook broccoli lightly... Steam it in a little liquid for 3 to 4 minutes until bright green, using a steamer so that it doesn't touch the cooking liquid.

- Blanch it for 20 to 30 seconds, no more. (Blanching apparently destroys the myrosinase)

- Eating a small piece of raw broccoli with your cooked broccoli to add back the enzyme.

- Frozen broccoli is no good... It has no active myrosinase.

- Add a tiny amount of daikon radish to frozen broccoli. This will add back the needed enzyme.

It turns out that broccoli sprouts are even better than regular, adult broccoli. These are three-to four-day-old broccoli plants that look like alfalfa, but taste like radishes.

No idea if that's a good thing or not

The sprouts boast up to 100 times more sulforaphane per unit of weight than a head of broccoli.

I have read these blogs, or tried to, and was both encouraged and disheartened. People really do want to be healthy and eat their broccoli correctly, which was great. On the other hand, it seemed like far too much work for the ordinary, non-OCD type person.

Thus, welcome big business.

In 2010, PharmAgra Labs Inc, a US chemical synthesis company discovered a method for synthesizing and stabilizing sulforaphane in a sugar lattice. The company branded the stabilized sulforaphane technology, Sulforadex®.

Focusing on academic research to prove its efficacy, they have concentrated on the activation of Nrf2; and the production of proteins with antioxidative, anti-inflammatory and cytoprotective qualities.

They haven't addressed any anti-aging effects directly that I know of, but they have looked at breast cancer, subarachnoid hemorrhage, prostate cancer, and multiple sclerosis.

Another trick to making sulforaphane more bioavailable has been the micro-encapsulation of sulforaphane by gelatin/gum arabic and gelatin/pectin complexes. This at least in the literature, has improved bioactivity.

Other companies have brought us BroccoPhane® and BroccoSinolate™ from Cyvex Nutrition, and BroccoPlus™ by Omega Protein Corporation. There is no indication of why these formulations might be better, but they do have good names.

• •

> *"Dietary supplement manufacturers may now combine the powerful properties of broccoli with BroccoSinolate™ and BroccoPhane™ for detoxification products, immune support products and antioxidant complexes," says Gilbert Gluck, president and CEO of Cyvex Nutrition.*

• •

The last and maybe the best idea goes back to the discoverer of all of this, Dr. Tony Talalay. He and his company have put out a product called Truebroc. I'm not sure if the name is supposed to be funny, true or even a bit ironic; they are packaging the base molecule, glucoraphanin, the one prior to its conversion into an active form. So, Truebroc is accurate, this really is the ingredient in broccoli. What it does not have, however, is the enzyme.

But the company isn't even trying to simulate the enzyme. They are banking on one simple realization: Your gut bacteria can actually convert the glucoraphanin to sulforaphane all by itself. It turns out you don't actually need the fancy enzyme. You, or the bacteria in your GI tract, already have it.

Thus, they are selling a capsule that is equivalent to 1 and one-fourth cups of broccoli. It offers nothing else... it's just easier than eating the actual vegetable.

So, do we need all of the fancy cooking strategies or specialized formulations? I don't have a magic eight ball, but the answer seems like we do not.

The irony in all of this is clear:

"When compared with other phytochemicals widely used in dietary supplements, sulforaphane is significantly more bioavailable than polyphenols such as curcumin, resveratrol and silymarin."[4]

So, it turns out that all of these folks have been trying to improve upon something that, in reality, wasn't really necessary after all.

Kaufmann Number: 3.2.0.1.0.2.0

CHAPTER 20:

QUERCETIN

Quercetin is presently what I consider one of the second tier supplements in terms of anti-aging. It may, however, be on the cusp of greatness. For example, it does do very important things such as being an antioxidant and an anti-inflammatory. In fact, it is the only one that decreases histamine release. As well, there are several properties that, if proven to be true, could catapult it into the prime category. At the moment however, the evidence remains scant. On the other hand, it would be unfair to keep it from you.

• •

"Quercetin is a polyphenolic compound with potent pleiotropic bioactivities including anti proliferative, anti-inflammatory, antioxidant, and immune system effects."[1]

"Quercetin exerts a large spectrum of biological effects: anti-inflammatory, anti-infectious, antioxidant, anticancer/ chemopreventive, neuroprotective, antihypertensive and glucose lowering properties have been reported."[2]

"It has been shown that quercetin possesses anti-atherogenic, anti-inflammatory, anticoagulative and anti-hypertensive properties."[3]

• •

Let's start at the beginning.

Quercetin hasn't been around in teas for thousands of years, it hasn't traveled the globe, and it hasn't saved the world from any plagues; but it has been sitting on the kitchen table forever, and someone finally decided to take a closer look.

Quercetin, aka (3,3,4,5,7- pentahydroxyfavone), is a plant-based substance, and is considered a polyphenol based on the molecular structure of having many attached phenol groups.

The greatest amount of quercetin is found in cappers (233 mg/100gm), raw yellow chili peppers (50 mg/100gm) and onions (22mg/100gm). In onions, the substance is mostly in the outer layers, thus avoid excessive peeling. Quercetin is present in some fruits as well, mostly in apple and mostly in the peel. It is also in black tea and white wine. Recall that resveratrol is also in red wine, so if you prefer the whites just tell your friends you are more interested in the quercetin effect.[4]

What does it do exactly?

Quercetin is marketed as a supplement for allergies, asthma, arthritis, gout, hypertension and neurodegenerative disorders.[4]

• •

"Similar to other polyphenols, reported beneficial effects of quercetin include effects on cardiovascular diseases, cancer, infections, inflammatory processes, gastrointestinal tract function, diabetes, and nervous system disorders."[5]

• •

Mitochondria / Energy Systems: Antioxidant

Like almost all of our life-enhancing supplements, quercetin is a powerful antioxidant, working both directly and indirectly.

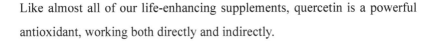

> *"Quercetin seems to be one of the most powerful flavonoids for protecting the body against reactive oxygen species."[6]*

However, in this instance, at high concentrations, it can actually become an oxidant itself and precipitate double-stranded DNA breaks. How much is too much? It's hard to say. In cell cultures, a low concentration of 1 nanoM was beneficial, but 100 nanoM was detrimental.[7] What this means in terms of human intake is difficult to determine.

Quercetin is also known to activate our own, endogenous antioxidants. Activating the Nrf2 (nuclear factor-like 2) pathway, it has significant control over the endogenous antioxidants that we have come to know and love: heme-oxygenate-1, glutamate cysteine ligase, glutathione S-transferase, glutathione peroxidase, superoxide dismutase, catalase, sulfiredoxin and thioredoxin.[5]

> *"Quercetin has been shown to counteract oxidative stress-induced cellular damage by activating the Nrf2-ARE pathway."[5]*

Pathways: Activates AMP Kinase

"AMPK is a serine /threonine protein kinase and is activated by several natural compounds, including resveratrol, epigallocatechin gallate, berberine, and quercetin."[8] This effect has been looked at in its role as having an effect on the treatment of obesity.

• •

" ...these data indicate that quercetin exerts anti-adipogenesis activity by activating the AMPK signal pathway in 3T3-L1 preadipocytes."[9]

• •

Quality Control: Proteasome Activator

As you may recall, protein production is key to cell survival. Unfortunately as we age, protein production declines. While the evidence in the literature is a little thin, quercetin has been labeled as a proteasome activator.

• •

"Quercetin and its derivative, quercetin caprylate, both proteasome activators with antioxidant activity, increase cellular life span, survival, and viability of HLF-1 primary human fibroblast... ... Strikingly, application of these compounds to senescent fibroblasts induces a rejuvenating effect."[7]

• •

Immune System / Security: Anti-inflammatory

Since 1977, scientists have been aware that quercetin blocks histamine release. If you recall, histamine is produced and then excreted by various cells in response to stress, which then further stimulates the inflammatory response. Histamine is responsible for that itching that drives you crazy.

Quercetin acts by inhibiting mast cell activation, and thus blocks the release of histamine. There is even a quercetin nasal spray that effectively treats sinusitis, allergic rhinitis and asthma. In fact, when compared to a popular asthma medication, cromolyn, (which is prescription) they had comparable results in terms of suppressing symptoms. Both compounds were equally able to block the histamine release, but quercetin was actually better at reducing levels of IL-8.[6]

Outside of histamine release, quercetin also reduces inflammatory cytokines. In human cell cultures, it specifically decreased IL-4, IL-6, IL-8, and IL-13.

• •

> *"The anti-inflammatory action of quercetin is caused by the inhibition of enzymes such as lipogenase, and the inhibition of inflammatory mediators. Quercetin affects immunity and inflammation by acting mainly on leukocytes and targeting many intracellular signaling kinases and phosphates, enzymes and membrane proteins ... "*[6]

• •

Individual Cell Health: Senolytic

This category is important, yet the evidence here is little thin at the moment (This is what could potentially catapult quercetin into the spotlight).

As we discussed in the chapter on cells, senescent cells tend to become malevolent over time. Once fully functioning, they devolve into bitter old men that incite unrest among their peers. As we have learned, these cells actually secrete inflammatory cytokines, aka SASPs or Senescence-Associated Secretory Phenotypes. It is thought that the accumulation of such cells leads to both local and systemic diseases. Thus, there is an ongoing search for agents that will selectively get rid of these senescent cells. In various studies, the removal of only 30% of such cells can demonstrate a dramatic improvement in age-related disease.

At the moment, there are only a few agents that are thought to be in this category, notably, dasatinib and quercetin. The two molecules seem to work better in conjunction than separately, but I don't recommend taking dasatinib if you don't have to. It is marketed as a chemotherapy drug for leukemia, *Sprycel*, and comes with a terrible list of side effects such as neutropenia, severe immune suppression, and pleural effusions.

Meanwhile, quercetin does show independent activity against human epithelial cells, as well as senescent bone marrow-derived mouse mesenchymal stem cells.

• •

> *"These data ...demonstrate that both Dasatinib and Quercetin are able to selectively kill senescent cells, albeit with distinct cell-type specificity."*[10]

• •

As I said, the evidence is a little lacking, but if quercetin can actually clear out senescent cells, then this becomes a huge deal.

• •

> *"Thus, interventions that reduce the burden of senescent cells could ameliorate age related disabilities and chronic diseases as a group."*[10]

• •

Inhibits Metabolism of Resveratrol

Quercetin inhibits CYP3A4, one of the enzymes that metabolizes substances in the liver. Thus it is possible that the effects of other supplements, especially resveratrol or medications may be effected as well.[11]

So, it seems like quercetin would be a reasonable addition to our arsenal. But, the question always arises: how much to take?

Currently, over the counter supplements range from 250 to 1500 mg, usually in the aglycone form. Very large doses, i.e., IV doses up to 3600 mg, can cause some kidney issues. A single dose of 1095 mg was shown to increase the plasma level three fold.

In some literature, the recommended dose is 1 gm/day.[5]

Given a normal western diet, between 15 to 40 mg of quercetin are generally consumed daily. One study demonstrated that you need at least 33 mg/day to see any cardiovascular improvements.

Realizing there is a huge difference between 33 mg and 1 gram, clearly no one really knows. Because, in reality, we are not treating an actual disease exactly, just aging.

Kaufmann Number: 0.3.1.2.2.2.0

CHAPTER 21:

EGCG OR EPIGALLOCATECHIN GALLATE - A CUP OF TEA?

Imbibing green tea is good for you; people have known this for thousands of years. In fact, we believe it was first used (roughly) in 3,000 BC, making it about 5,000 years old. Originally brewed by the Chinese, it was brought to Japan by Buddhist monks a thousand or so years later.

The health benefits of tea were described in 1211 by a Japanese Zen priest by the name of Yeisai. The book, "Kitcha-Yojoki," translates to Tea and Health promotion.

Years later, somewhere between 1630 and 1714, a doctor during the Edo period in Japan named Ekiken Kaibara, also wrote about it in a book entitled "Yojokun" or Lessons for Health Promotion. He however proclaimed that the drinking of green tea was not beneficial as it led to weight loss.[1]

Clearly issues with obesity have changed over time ▸

Green tea is brewed from the leaves and buds of the plant *Camellia sinensis*. Importantly, it is not fermented. Black tea, meanwhile, comes from the same plant and is fermented, while oolong tea is semi-fermented.

So, the great Chinese have been drinking this wonderful elixir for a zillion (plus or minus) years. This of course, in today's world is no longer good enough. So, let the dissection begin.

Green tea extract is composed of innumerable components:

- The major component is EGCG or Epigallocatechin gallate… somewhere between 18% and up. One paper, for example, puts it somewhere between 50-80%.
- 11.6% gallocatechin 3-o-gallate
- 4.6% epicatechin 3-o-gallate
- 15% epigallocatechin
- 14.8% gallocatechin
- 7% epicatechin
- 3.5% catechin

Realizing all of these sound roughly the same, the reality is that they are all very close. The other reality is the only one that is actually important is the first: Epigallocatechin gallate, aka EGCG.

Other than being good tea, or even great if you're a fan, why are we talking about tea?

In addition to the ability to act as a neutralizing agent of excessive ROS, EGCG exerts antioxidant, anti-inflammatory and anti-tumorigenic effects."[2]

• •

"This ability is mostly attributed to their antioxidant, radical scavenging, metal chelating, anti-carcinogenic, anti-apoptotic and anti-inflammatory properties."[4]

"EGCG was found to exert profound anti-inflammatory, antioxidant, anti-infective, anticancer, antiangiogenic, and chemopreventative effects."[3]

"In the last decade, green tea polyphenols, particularly its active component EGCG, has gained a lot of attention as a potential therapeutic agent for preventing neurodegenerative, inflammatory diseases and cancer mainly due to their beneficial effects on human health."[4]

It has been "found to be helpful with: cardiovascular diseases, neurodegenerative diseases, cancer, inflammatory diseases, metabolic diseases, obesity and AGING."[4]

• •

Enough said, let's take a closer look.

Assuming you're a rat that has been drinking tea since infancy ▶ Let's answer the big question first. Can EGCG actually help you live longer? The answer is a resounding yes....

In a lifetime rat study, the median lifespan for the controls were 92.5 weeks. The addition of EGCG increased this to 105 weeks. At the end of the study, as compared to the controls, the study group had less damage to the kidneys and liver, had decreased NF-κβ and increased SIRT1.[5]

To the list!

DNA / Information Systems: Epigenetic Modifier

As we have mentioned previously, the field of epigenetics and aging is fairly new. We know that EGCG effects the epigenetic footprint, but exactly how this occurs is a little hazy. It is however, included in our elite epigenetic diet.

What exactly does it do? Biochemically, EGCG inhibits DNA methylation and inhibits histone deacetylation activity.[6]

• •

"EGCG binds to the active site residue of the DNMT1 to directly inhibit activity. This prevents methylation of newly synthesized DNA and ultimately leads to expression of previously silenced genes."[6]

• •

In a skin cancer model, we know that EGCG acts as an epigenetic regulator that suppresses DNA methylation in a time and dose-dependent manner. This somehow translates into a better outcome in terms of the cancer.

Mitochondria / Energy Systems: Antioxidant

As we have now seen many times, to be part of the exclusive anti-aging protocol, the compound must offer some antioxidant qualities. Ideally, there might be both direct free radical scavenging and a secondary, indirect production of endogenous antioxidant enzymes. In both regards, EGCG does not disappoint.

In the direct sense, EGCG has been reported to be more effective as a radical scavenger when compared to vitamin E and C.[4]

• •

"Green tea polyphenols are biological antioxidants with radical scavenging properties. Among the green tea polyphenol family, EGCG and ECG are the most potent radical scavengers."[4]

• •

In a culture of human stem cells, EGCG also was found to be effective via the nuclear factor erythroid 2-related factor (Nrf2) mechanism, stimulating the downstream antioxidant genes.[2]

Recall that Nrf2 plays an important role in the cellular antioxidant defense system by activating the expression of multiple antioxidant and detoxifying genes, such as superoxide dismutase, heme oxygenate 1, and glutathione S-transferase.

As icing on the cake, in a double-blinded, placebo controlled human study, after treatment with EGCG, the total antioxidant status was much higher. As well, acting as an anti-inflammatory, serum TNF-α and C-reactive protein were significantly lower.[1]

Pathways: Activates AMP Kinase

"AMPK is a serine /threonine protein kinase and is activated by several natural compounds, including resveratrol, epigallocatechin gallate, berberine, and quercetin."[8] In this category, we know not only that EGCG can activate AMP Kinase, but also how it does what it does.

"In defining the mechanism by which EGCG activates AMPK, we found that the EGCG activation of AMPK was mediated by the Ca+ / calmodulin - dependent protein kinase kinase (CaMKK)."[9]

Quality Control: Autophagy

If you recall from previous chapters, autophagy is the recycling system of the cell. Old or warn out proteins, lipids and organelles get degraded via the lysosomal pathway so that new products can be made in their place. You may remember as well, this is highly correlated to improved health and health span.

Multiple studies have demonstrated that EGCG promotes autophagy, especially in the liver.

• •

"Here we show that EGCG increases hepatic autophagy by promoting the formation of autophagosomes, increasing lysosomal acidification, and stimulating autophagic flux in hepatic cells and in vivo."[10]

• •

The effects of EGCG on autophagy also seem to be tissue specific. It is known to promote autophagy in macrophages and endothelial cells in addition to liver cells. Much like melatonin, however, EGCG seems to decrease autophagy in human retinal pigment epithelial cells. No one has any idea why this is so, but it does.

Immune System / Security

In this category, there is significant evidence demonstrating the anti-inflammatory properties of EGCG. It has been shown repeatedly in many tissue types to inhibit TNF-α, IL-1β, IL-6, C-reactive protein and COX-2. It can also mitigate the release of MMP-3 and MMP-9 from macrophages.[11,12]

Individual Cell Health: Modulates Output of Stem Cells

As will be discussed below, EGCG has an osteo-inductive effect on stem cells, meaning the cells are steered into making bone cells versus any other cell.

Waste Management: AGE Reduction

While it is not uncommon for many of our substances to lower blood sugar, very few of them have actually been proven scientifically to lower the levels of AGEs.

It's hard to find something that you aren't looking for!

Therefore, in yet another study of overfed, obese rats, the treatment group was given EGCG for 17 weeks. The agent significantly reduced weight gain, plasma glucose, the insulin level and both the liver and kidney weights. Importantly, it also decreased the levels of AGEs, and even the expression of their receptors, the RAGEs.[13]

• •

"Supplementation of a high fat diet with dietary EGCG significantly reduced weight gain, plasma glucose, insulin level, liver and kidney weight. EGCG administration also decreased the levels of AGEs in both plasma and liver while inhibiting the receptor for AGE (RAGE) expression."[13]

• •

Weight Loss

The effect on weight loss has been known for hundreds, if not thousands of years. The complicating fact, however, is that humans want instant results and they don't follow directions very well. For example, when it became known that green tea was a weight-loss adjuvant, people went nuts. They drank 10 to 15 cups a day, and tried to shed too many pounds too quickly.

In human studies, results trying to examine this have been conflicting. The reality is that by drinking about 2 cups a day, you can burn up about 100 extra calories in a 24 hour period. This isn't earth shattering, but it shouldn't be. It takes time to put on extra weight, so it should take a little time to get rid of it.

On the other hand, it is much easier to control rats, especially fat ones.

It has been clearly shown that the administration of EGCG to obese rats increased the percentage of their fat-free mass. Conveniently, it also increased bone mineral density and bone strength, and it decreased pro-inflammatory cytokines, including TNF-α.

Speaking of bone mineral density and strength…

Bone

As we have talked about before, osteoporosis is a severe disease characterized by decreased bone mineral density and degraded bone fiber structure. It is especially harsh on postmenopausal women, when the number of pathological fractures increase significantly.

In humans, several epidemiological studies have reported an association of consumption of green tea with reduced risk of osteoporosis. This is not pure evidence however, as self-reporting of diet and activity is rarely accurate.

However, in human mesenchymal stem cells, i.e., sitting in a laboratory on a plate, EGCG exerts an osteoinductive effect on MSC's, as evidenced by increased bone-forming enzyme activity, the upregulated expression osteogenic genes and the formation of bone-like nodules. Furthermore, the effect of EGCG on osteoporosis is dose-dependent.[14]

Therefore, for at least culture human stem cells, EGCG is effective as a pro-osteogenic agent in stem cells. Hopefully, this translates into better bones for the rest of us.

Brain

The brain is a tricky organ. The good news is that EGCG is able to cross the blood brain barrier, and can deliver relief to a stressed system. In fact, studies both at the cellular level up to practical behaviors have all demonstrated real benefits.

On the cellular level, "green tea polyphenols are known to possess neuroprotective and neuro-rescue action. In particular, EGCG has been shown to increase cell viability, decrease reactive oxygen species and expression levels of endoplasmic reticulum stress markers and apoptotic markers."[4]

As well, adult hippocampal neurogenesis is a unique form of neural circuit plasticity that is present throughout life. This allows for a lifetime (hopefully) of making new memories or learning new things. In yet another rat study, EGCG was shown to enhance adult hippocampal nerve generation.[15]

In terms of practical brain utilization, both small mammal and human studies have shown an improvement in learning and other brain activities. As well, many studies have demonstrated that EGCG exerts protective effects against seemingly eventual age-related cognitive declines and neurodegenerative diseases.[15]

In rats, the long-term administration of EGCG also reported significant improvement in spacial cognitive learning ability.[4]

Epidemiological studies, meanwhile, have shown a clear, inverse association between green tea consumption and cognitive dysfunction in dementia, Alzheimer's disease and Parkinson's disease.[15]

• •

"Extensive research on EGCG have brought into light their potential to promote healthy aging by improving the morphological and functional alterations that occur in a natural aging brain, their

ability to suppress cognitive dysfunction, increase learning ability and reduce oxidative damage in the brain."[4]

• •

Warts

On a bizarre side note, I discovered that in 2006, a green tea extract was approved as a prescription drug for the topical treatment of genital and anal warts.[3]

It is very clear that green tea and more specifically, EGCG, carry innumerable health benefits. Once again, you can either choose to have a cup of tea, or resort to concentrated capsules.

There are about 70 to 90 mg of EGCG per cup of green tea. By comparison, the average capsule has between 400 to 500 mg.

The highest blood levels peak at about 1.5 hours, and can be found in your urine for up to about 15 hours.

Mild side effects are reported by those who have taken a bit too much, including nausea and heartburn.

Kaufmann Number: 2.2.1.2.1.1.2

CHAPTER 22:

ASTRAGALUS RADIX MEMBRANACEUS

Despite sounding like a Roman general, the roots of astragalus are actually Chinese, and the plant is infamous for increasing one's life force or Qi. I'll reiterate for the sake of the skimmers out there, it will increase your life force. Sounds impressive…right?

How many substances can actually do this? Not many!

In fact, out of the two thousand astragalus plant species, only two have medicinal properties and only one has this special capability. Thus, knowing the full name of our newest ally is important as it should be properly recognized.

Astragalus R. Membranaceus has a very long history. It has been used in Chinese medicine for over 2,000 years, and as I mentioned, it has the lofty goal of strengthening the Qi. Literally translated as breath, air or gas, it has been known to mean the energy flow or life force.

Coming from the western world, I'm not completely sure what this all means. However, it's hard to argue with anything that can increase my life force. It even seems like the "force may be with me."

When imbibed as a tea or tonic, the substance is supposed to increase stamina, strength and vitality. Reportedly, it guards also against physical, mental and even emotional stress.

All good things! ▶

More specifically in the historical, medical literature, it is used to treat wounds, fever, allergies, chronic fatigue, stomach ulcers, uterine bleeding and even loss of appetite. It has been reported to offer liver protection, act as an anti-inflammatory and antioxidant, and lower blood sugar.

The plant itself is endogenous to Northern China, Mongolia and Korea, although presently, it is mostly farmed in China. As well the only component of the species utilized is derived from the roots of four-year-old plants.

Once upon a time, the Chinese were content to enjoy their Qi without question. We however, in the western world, have elected to dissect this magical elixir.

It turns out that the astragalus plant is composed of over 100 individual, active chemical components including flavonoids, saponins, polysaccharides, and amino acids. The actual concentrations of each however, vary by the region in which they were grown, and when they were harvested.

Within the saponin family, we find the several interesting molecules, including cycloastrogenol, astragaloside IV, cyclocephaloside, and cyclocanthoside. In the flavonoid family, we find our now familiar friend, quercetin. In addition, there are about 20 different amino acids, and more than 20 trace elements such as scandium, cobalt, copper, selenium, iron, manganese, and zinc.[1]

Because there are so many different substances in astragalus, we are going to take a peak at just a few of them.

Cycloastrogenol

The most notable component isolated from astragalus at the moment is cycloastrogenol. Following the discovery of telomeres and their important connection to aging, there was a grand search for any compound that might augment telomere length, or at the very least, preserve it over time. The answer arrived in the form of cycloastrogenol.

The compound was first studied by the Geron corporation, but then exclusive rights were secured by TA Sciences in 2002 (per their website). The company developed it as a product called TA-65 (very secretive) and introduced it to a select market in 2007. In late 2013 and again in 2014, another company, RevGenetics, determined that TA-65 was actually cycloastrogenol and released the information to the public. So, the secret was no longer a secret. Presently, you can purchase either, although both are pretty expensive.

Does it work? Can it increase telomeres?

First, a bit of review.

If you recall, telomeres are the protective caps at the end of our DNA. Every time a cell divides, the telomere length gets truncated. They also get shorter in response to cellular stresses. In some cells, peripheral lymphocytes and stem cells for example, there is an enzyme, telomerase, that can produce more DNA. It simply adds more base pairs to the end. Unfortunately, this enzyme isn't in all cells, and importantly, even in cells where it exists, it is not sufficient to maintain telomere length over time.

The association between length of life and length of telomeres is pretty strong. What's lacking however, is the evidence that artificially lengthening the telomeres actually works to elongate life. Regardless, there is a lot of money and a lot of hope banking on this idea.

The first place to generally test these ideas are of course in mice. Thus, a study "indicated that TA-65 treatment resulted in telomerase-dependent elongation of short telomeres and rescue of associated DNA damage, thus demonstrating that TA-65 is capable of action through the telomerase pathway."[2] (This of course was written when the mystery substance was TA-65.)

As well, mice studies demonstrated that the female-treated mice did better overall in terms of certain health span indicators such as glucose tolerance, higher bone density, and better skin fitness.[2]

Of note, another set of mice treated with oral cycloastrogenol for seven days were significantly less depressed.[3]

Clearly they were suffering from a lack of Qi!

Finches were another species treated with TA-65. Not only were their telomeres longer, but their feathers grew faster.[4]

Rising up the chain of study models, the next thing to examine are human cell cultures. In this particular study, cells from HIV-1 infected persons were treated with the substance.

"In this study, we demonstrate that TAT2 (cycloastrogenol) can transiently activate telomerase, slow telomere loss, increase replicative capacity, and importantly, enhance immune function in CD8+T lymphocytes from HIV-1 infected persons."[5]

They concluded that "telomerase activators, such as TAT2 (cycloastrogenol) may constitute a novel class of therapeutic agents which improve immune function at a fundamental, cellular aging level."[5]

Therefore, the cells not only survived, but showed signs of improvement. Next up, real people.

Published in 2016, 117 healthy people aged 53 to 87 were given TA-65 (250u). Over the course of one year, there was a significant increase in the telomeres of the treatment group; (530 +/-180 bp's) vs the control group that lost length (290 +/-100 bp's).[6]

Another interesting study looked at the effect of cycloastrogenol on vision. This was based on a previous study that had connected telomeric length with Age-Related Macular Degeneration.

Thirty-eight patients, ranging in age from 52 to 83 (mean of 71), took the adjuvant for one year. They didn't have to wait that long however, there was obvious improvement at 6 months, and it maintained at one year. This was based not only on perception of vision, but measurement of macular function.[7]

In other studies looking to see what cycloastrogenol could do, it was found to be quite active in wound healing. Compared to the other saponins, cycloastrogenol was discovered to be the most remarkable in vivo wound healing agent. Specifically, it demonstrated greater cell density, a more regular organized dermis, and more newly formed blood vessels (rat study).[8]

The other important concern connected with the idea of increasing telomeres is the question of cancer. Many types of cancer are difficult to eradicate as these cells have significant amounts of telomerase.

Therefore, these cells just keep multiplying despite chemotherapy. People have feared that the addition of cycloastrogenol might therefore be cancer promoting. The good news is that, to date, there has been no evidence of this.

• •

> *"Importantly, treatment with TA-65 did not show any detectable negative secondary effects, including no increase in the incidence of cancer."*[2]

• •

In addition, there are several other agents that have been found to increase telomeres - including sulforaphane, carnosine, N-acetyl-cystein and Vitamin D. These do not, however, come even close to cycloastrogenol.[9]

Astragaloside IV

The bastard cousin, astragaloside IV, unfortunately cannot compete in terms of telomere enhancement. It does however, have other ways of increasing your Qi.

Interestingly, it seems to be particularly good at neuron growth and repair.

"In the central nervous system, astragaloside IV has contributed to nerve repair….accelerated axon growth in mouse hippocampus, prevented neuronal atrophy and memory loss…"[10]

"Astragaloside IV promotes neural regeneration or prevents neural injury through various mechanisms."[10]

It also demonstrates a few more typical anti-aging activities: inhibiting inflammation, oxidation, and apoptosis, and exerting immunoregulatory effects.

Astragalus Polysaccharides

This substance mostly demonstrates anti-inflammatory properties. Notably, it blocks TNF-α with the downstream effects of reduced cytokines including NF-κβ, ICAM (intercellular adhesion molecule-1) and VCAM (vascular cell adhesion molecule-1), as determined in human vascular endothelial cells.[11]

Whereas there are a zillion other substances in the astragalus plant, few have been as avidly studied. Therefore, you have several choices. You can either partake of the entire root, or simply utilize it's components.

Either way, there was a great warning on one of the Chinese herbal websites that you may find interesting. Astragalus was not to be taken by anyone with excess Qi. So, if you happen to have excess Qi (I'm not sure who might fall into this category…perhaps a Jedi knight)…beware, it could be dangerous.

Kaufmann Number: 3.0.0.0.2.1.0

CHAPTER 23:

MELATONIN

Melatonin means many things to many people. Most of the time, it's what you take at night when you can't sleep. No one really seems to know what it actually is, but it certainly aids in sleeping and eliciting vivid, colorful dreams.

So, what is it really? There are actually two answers to this question. For the science folks out there, it is an ancient molecule, technically an endogenously produced indolamine, N-acetyl-5- methoxytryptamin.

Melatonin exists in almost every cell type there is, from single-celled organisms, to plants, and especially in us. Certainly, it isn't there to help plants sleep. So, why is it there? The hypothesis presently is that it developed 3.2ish billion years ago as an antioxidant.[1] Why? Because scientists have identified it in very ancient organisms, specifically purple, non-sulfur bacteria and cyanobacteria that were most likely the precursors to mitochondria and chloroplasts. These were the cells that were later engulfed by the larger, energy-seeking cells way back when. These scientists also believe that melatonin is produced in the mitochondria of cells even today, as a remnant of their heritage.

Melatonin was first identified in 1917 in reptiles, and was thought to be the reason the animals could alter their skin color. In 1958 at Yale, it was isolated from bovine pineal gland (cow brain) and named for its ability to lighten skin of experimental animals.

In the mid-1970s, scientists discovered the circadian nature of melatonin in mammals, and it wasn't until 1993 that its antioxidant qualities were realized.

In the quest to make a dollar, melatonin was patented as an over the counter sleep aid in 1995 to a Dr. Wurtman at MIT.

The reality, however, is that melatonin has been around forever; it can be found almost everywhere you look, and can do some extraordinary things.

Not just to help you sleep!

For example, melatonin is in very common foods; including cherries, bananas, pineapples, oranges, grapes, rice, olive oil, wine and beer.

Another good reason to drink wine!

It was also thought at one time to be produced only in the pineal gland in the mammalian brain, but more recently it was noted to be produced in many places in mammals; especially the retina, the GI tract, platelets, bone marrow cells and of course, in the skin.

As a molecule, melatonin is both water and fat soluble, or amphiphilic, which means that it has the ability to pass though and into almost all cellular and sub-cellular barriers. I picture it as a general overseer; floating around to make sure all is well. Where it has limited access or needs a little assistance, there are two melatonin receptors, M1 and M2 (of course) to facilitate its actions.

The other thing you need to know is that over a lifetime, the concentrations of melatonin changes. During the first two weeks of life, there is a small but detectable amount of melatonin in the bloodstream, but there is no nocturnal pattern. This eventual evening rise begins at about three months, probably when babies first start sleeping through the night.

Unless you are an extremely lucky parent!

The highest nocturnal rise occurs between the ages of 4 to 7, and then declines again until puberty. Unfortunately, as we all know, life goes down hill sometime after puberty, as does the concentrations of melatonin.[5]

• •

"Melatonin production, amplitude and its pulsatile release from the pineal gland decrease upon aging."[2]

• •

I said there were two answers to the question about what melatonin really is. The second answer is much more fun than the first. You see, I believe that melatonin is the molecular equivalent of Mary Poppins.

You may not remember exactly who Mary Poppins is, so allow me to remind you. She was, of course, the magical nanny to the Bank's children, who required a little guidance as well as a bit of fun. She told them when to go to bed at night, but made sure their dreams were magical. She didn't always do what you thought a good nanny ought to, but her ways always worked out in the end. In essence, she did what she had to do, even if you failed to understand the why or the how.

She was present, as is melatonin, in small children, and disappears a bit when we are adults. But, as we need more answers over time, we turn to her once again.

• •

"In view of these findings, melatonin is not a hormone in the classic sense, but functions as a cell protector and also as an antioxidant."[3]

"Melatonin seems to be involved in the maintenance of a healthy state of metabolic regulation."[3]

"Melatonin provides both in vivo and in vitro protection at the level of the cell membrane, mitochondria, and nucleus, partly due to its free-radical scavenging and antioxidant properties."[4]

• •

What exactly does melatonin do that is so special? It does a plethora of things:

"This indole plays an important role in many physiological processes including circadian entrainment, blood pressure regulation, seasonal reproduction, ovarian physiology, immune function, etc."[5]

"Administration of melatonin was unanimously reported to reduce the signs of metabolic syndrome, such as hyperglycemia, dyslipidemia, hyperinsulinemia, insulin resistance, weight gain, and hypertension"…in normal rats fed a high fat diet, diabetic fatty rats, and even aging rats.[3]

"Melatonin exerts a broad spectrum of effects on physiological functions of relevance to aging, such as metabolic sensing, mitochondrial modulation and presumably also proliferation, antioxidation protection of biomolecules and sub cellular structures, in particular, mitochondria."[3]

Lets look a bit closer at some of our nanny's effects:

DNA / Information Systems: Epigenetic Modification

As we have seen, it is fairly straightforward to determine if a molecule is an epigenetic modifier. Unfortunately, it is a little more difficult to determine if these changes are beneficial or not. Therefore, most studies examining epigenetic effects have tended to focus on cancer, as it is easier to determine outcome. Thus, melatonin falls into the same category as most of our modifiers; we know it adjusts the DNA and we know it fights against cancer. What is does to aging remains a guess.

• •

"Melatonin causes epigenetic effects against cancer cells by modulating with DNA methylation and histone acetylation pathways."[2]

"Melatonin can restore liver histone deacetylase, DNA methyltransferase activity, and DNA methylation."[2]

• •

On an interesting note, long-term shift works end up with hypomethylation of the CLOCK genes and hyper methylation of CRY2.

Mitochondria / Energy Systems: Antioxidant

As you have probably realized, to be included in the anti-aging regime, there must be a contribution in the antioxidant category; and melatonin is no exception.

Melatonin is, in fact both a powerful direct and indirect antioxidant.

• •

"Regarding UV-induced oxidative damage, it has been shown that melatonin is a strong scavenger against UV-induced formation of ROS, and even biologically more potent in this capacity than vitamin C or Vitamin E."[6]

• •

It has been shown to be directly protective in many tissues, including pancreatic cells, brain cells and even the discs between your vertebrae.

• •

"Melatonin displays a protective effect against reactive oxygen species (ROS) generation in pancreatic β-cells, which are easily susceptible to oxidative stress."[2]

• •

Melatonin also upregulates the gene expression and activity of our now favorite protective enzymes, including "Cu/Zn-superoxide dismutase, Mn-superoxide dismutase, catalase and glutathione peroxidase."[6]

Pathways: Indirect Control Over the Sirtuin Pathway

Circadian rhythms exert control over the sirtuin pathways, and alas, melatonin controls the circadian rhythms.

Melatonin, otherwise known as the "hormone of darkness," is primarily secreted at night and controls, and is itself controlled, by the light and dark cycles.

If you recall from the sirtuin section of the pathway chapter, the circadian rhythms are a continuous battle between two day time proteins (CLOCK/ BMAL1) and two night time proteins (PERS/CRYs). This oscillation in turn regulates innumerable other oscillatory factors in the body, including the production of NAD^+ and the sirtuins.

That's when we take everything for granted... ▶ We take the circadian cycle for granted most of the time, especially when we are young.

When we are sleeping well, there is no reason to think about the need for sleep; but, as we age, there is the seemingly inevitable shift in the cycle whereby older people just can't sleep.

Unfortunately, this is more than just an annoying problem. Countless secondary functions rely upon the circadian cycle, and the body does not do well when it becomes interrupted. In fact, it is well established that the control of metabolism, the oxidative stress response, as well as DNA repair are intrinsically linked to sleep patterns.[2]

In fact, failure of the sleep cycle is known to contribute to the onset of premature aging.

• •

"Circadian clock dysfunction contributes to aging and age-related pathologies."[2]

• •

The other thing that occurs as the clock shifts is an alteration in the DNA. Epigenetic changes through histone acetylation can then affect a slew of secondary issues including a depressed immune system.

Even in younger people that alter their own circadian rhythms for whatever reasons, their health is negatively effected. In fact, workers that have abnormal circadian cycles secondary to abnormal shifts have an increase in neurodegeneration, metabolic syndromes and even cancer.

Quality Control: Autophagy

If you recall from the chapter on quality control, autophagy is when a cell decides to reprocess old and worn out proteins and structures. The ability to recycle is key to cells that are longer lived, especially neurons. As we well know:

"Macroautophagy is also a factor that is repressed during aging."[2]

Because Mary Poppins seems to have a mind of her own and can never be truly straight forward, melatonin as well has varying effects on autophagy.

"Melatonin can act as either pro-or anti-autophagy. It depends on the stage of autophagy. In normal physiological condition, melatonin will help or activate autophagy for cell survival. On the other hand, when cells are exposed to ROS or toxic agents, autophagy (excessive levels) will shift to autophagic cell death. In this state, melatonin exhibits protective effects to inhibit excessive lavages of autophagy."[2]

Immune Systems / Security: Anti-inflammatory

The second requisite category is that of staving off inflammation; and again, this is one of those instances where the nanny knows best. At times, melatonin increases the inflammatory response, and at other times, she suppresses it.

• •

"While melatonin exerts anti-inflammatory effects in various models of experimental high-grade inflammation, it has been reported to act, under basal conditions, as an immune enhancer and, thereby, as a potentially pro inflammatory and pro-oxidant agent."[3]

"Melatonin acts as a buffer for the immune system, displaying stimulant effects under basal or immunosuppressive conditions, and acting as an anti-inflammatory signal in situations where there is an exacerbated immune response."[4]

• •

But first, let's review the immune system a bit. The changes normally observed as we age may be primarily regarded as a process of deterioration because the aging immune system is less able to cope with infections.

At the same time, the senescent immune system becomes misdirected with an enhanced tendency toward inflammatory responses, autoimmune diseases, and cancer. Therefore, what we require here is a moderator. Something that can up regulate the infection fighting ability, while down regulating the negative aspects. Clearly, Mary Poppins is needed here; and amazingly enough, melatonin has the ability to do both, under the appropriate conditions.

• •

"This should not be regarded as a contradiction, because the immune system itself, in its remarkable complexity, comprises mechanisms for both types of action, as damping is required for avoiding overshooting reactions and for the process of healing."[3]

• •

In an example of when limiting the immune response is helpful, we turn once again to tortured rats. In a treadmill exercise where rats were run to exhaustion, the activity was noted to precipitate the overproduction of free radicals and inflammatory cytokines. After turning up the speed and the angle of inclination, eventually the rats fell off and were decapitated. Luckily (at least for us), those rats that were given melatonin prior to the event demonstrated a decrease in muscle concentrations of IL-1β (35%), TNF-α (13%), and IL-6 (48%).[7]

The thought was that "melatonin treatment may reverse the skeletal muscle inflammation and oxidative stress induced by strenuous exercise. These effects can help improve the recovery of athletes after exhaustive exercise."[7]

Thus, for anyone exercising, a bit of melatonin can make everything a bit better.

Just like a spoonful of sugar

In obesity models, fat rats fed very high fat diets in general, have increased markers of inflammatory cytokines. Remarkably, melatonin is able to normalize the altered biochemical pro-inflammatory profile. Specifically, melatonin decreased the augmented circulation levels of IL-1β, IL-6, TNF-α, and CRP.[4]

Individual Cell Health: Mesenchymal Stem Cell Effect

What are mesenchymal stem cells? Just in case you have forgotten, they are cells that can differentiate into a variety of unique cell types, such as osteoblasts, osteoclasts, chondrocytes, various blood cells, and adipocytes.

As the body ages, for whatever the reason, mesenchymal stem cells preferentially become fat cells instead of more useful cells like osteoblasts.

It is yet another reason we become fat when we age

The good news in this category is that melatonin alters this outcome; in the presence of melatonin, mesenchymal stem cells are more likely to become osteoblasts or bone-producing cells than fat cells.

• •

"Accumulating amounts of evidence suggests that melatonin affects osteoblast differentiation."[8]

"Recent studies have shown that melatonin affects bone formation through enhancing osteogenic differentiation. Melatonin treatment can prevent osteoporosis in ovariectomized rats and increase the volume of newly formed cortical bone of femora in mice."[8]

"Topical application of melatonin was found to accelerate osteointegration of dental implants and bone implants in Beagle dog and rabbit models."[8]

• •

It turns out that melatonin not only helps bone, but it helps the stem cells that are responsible for tooth growth as well.

Modulates Body Weight

In this category, there is only one effect. Melatonin absolutely helps to control weight gain and fat content.

In fact, if you remove anyone's pineal gland, thus reducing the amount of circulating melatonin, that individual will gain weight. If you return the melatonin, they subsequently lose the weight.

It is unclear if this effect has to do directly with melatonin, or an alteration in the circadian cycle. However, a disruption in the sleep/awake cycle is directly correlated to the development of obesity; and rotating shift work is associated with many components of metabolic syndrome.

Going in the other direction, a single daily administration of melatonin to middle-aged rats decreases their visceral fat.[9]

Thus, melatonin appears to carry an enormous and beneficial set of properties that can only help us as we age.

• •

"This chief secretory product of the pineal gland is now recognized to also exert numerous additional functions which range from free radical scavenging and DNA repair via immunomodulation, body weight control and the promotion of wound healing to the coupling of environmental cues to circadian clock gene expression and the modulation of secondary endocrine signaling."[6]

In fact, it has been called: "Nature's most versatile biological signal"[6]

• •

Let's see what it can do on the organ level.

Skin

In was known early on that melatonin was involved in the skin, thus the name of the substance; but it wasn't recognized until relatively recently that melatonin was actually produced in the skin as well.

• •

> *"Thus, the skin, the largest organ of the mammalian body, which engages in very complex, major endocrine activities has joined the growing number of mammalian tissues that operate as extra-pineal sites of melatonin synthesis."[6]*

• •

In other species that are renown for their skins and furs, this has been readily recognized. For example, melatonin can alter wool and cashmere production. Specifically, it can effect the development and frequency of pelage cycling, seasonal molting and even coat color.[6]

For people, melatonin is now thought to be extremely beneficial in treating skin problems such as photo damage, chronic skin inflammation and most signs of skin aging. Because concentrations in the skin fall as we age and oral supplementation doesn't reach ample concentrations in the skin, a topical melatonin is recommended.

Brain

As per usual, the brain suffers the most from disease secondary to oxidative stress and its high requirements for energy and oxygen.

As the decline of melatonin is quite prominent with age, it has been proposed that this is one of the primary contributing factors for the development of age-associated neurodegenerative diseases.[10]

As such, there have been innumerable studies looking at the supplementation of melatonin in the aging brain.

It turns out that melatonin is extremely beneficial. It has been shown to improve memory, improve cognitive function, and improve motor skills.

• •

"Melatonin may improve memory processes during aging through SIRT1 and circadian modulation because melatonin increased hippocampal SIRT1 level and improved cognitive functions in total sleep deprivation models. Moreover, memory formation is also controlled by circadian regulation."[2]

• •

"Chronic melatonin treatment improved learning and memory in a mouse model of brain deterioration."[11]

In an unrelated mouse model where a diabetic-like state was induced by D-galactose, the control group was found to have elevated levels of free oxygen radicals, AGE deposition and high numbers of receptors for the AGE molecules in the brain. The chronic administration of melatonin attenuated the memory impairment, synaptic dysfunction, the ROS and oxidative stress, the neuroinflammation, and the neurodegeneration.[11]

In another interesting model of how melatonin can save your brain, it turns out that: "Melatonin protects against neuronal cell death from methamphetamine toxicity."[2]

I'm extremely kidding... The lawyers would kill me! ▶ Thus, if you feel like a little meth on Friday night, pre-medicate with melatonin.

Bone

As I mentioned earlier in the mesenchymal stem cell section, melatonin is very good for the bones. There are probably several reasons for this (For a quick review, remember that osteoclasts destroy bone and osteoblasts rebuild it).

First, melatonin directly effects the actions of osteoblasts and osteoclasts. There are numerous studies documenting that melatonin increases pre-osteoblast and osteoblast proliferation. It also inhibits the differentiation of osteoclasts.[5]

Thus, less cells are around to destroy, with more cells that can rebuild and remodel.

Melatonin also promotes the expression of type I collagen, up regulates bone marker proteins, and stimulates the formation of mineralized matrix in these cells.[5]

Thus, much of the bone formation process is enhanced under the guidance of melatonin.

In a rabbit study of tibial bone implants with and without melatonin, it is not surprising that "Melatonin regenerated the width and length of cortical bone around implants in tibia of rabbits more quickly than around control implants without the addition of melatonin."[12]

As melatonin levels decline sharply after menopause, and osteoporosis rises dramatically, there is reason to believe that melatonin supplementation could be beneficial as a treatment. Presently, there are many people working hard to sort this out.

Sperm Quality[13]

This falls under the 'not my problem, but interesting nonetheless' category.

There is some evidence that infertile men have issues with their sperm, secondary to increased oxidative stress and possible DNA damage.

Thus, a group of infertile men were given a daily dose of 6 mg oral melatonin. After 45 days, there was a significant improvement noted in their sperm quality.

Similar studies have been conducted on infertile women as well, that were also treated with melatonin. These ladies demonstrated improved oocyte health and an increased pregnancy rate.

Exercise

It seems to be common knowledge that exercise at every age is good for you; but in a very telling study, even older, well-conditioned, trained rats experienced less benefit than if they were supplemented with melatonin.

It turns out that in order to see a reduced body mass, a higher gain in physical capacity, a decrease in triglycerides and an improved response to glucose, both exercise and melatonin were necessary.[9]

As well, the melatonin treatment was able to restore the mitochondrial quality and oxidative function. It considerably improved the physical performance induced by aerobic exercise training as well as in an endurance test.

In other words, "the muscle metabolic effect of the training protocol was only present in animals that were previously treated with melatonin."[9]

The take-home message was such...

"The present study demonstrates the importance of the therapeutic use of melatonin as a way to improve the beneficial responses induced by regular exercise in aging individuals, promoting a better quality of life and a healthier aging process."[9]

So, there it is. Melatonin is far much more than just a sleeping aid; it's a rejuvenation aid. Just ask Mary Poppins!

Kaufmann Number: 2.2.1.2.2.2.0

CHAPTER 24:

PYRIDOXAMINE

Many of the agents we have encountered so far seem to have a deep repertoire. They can scavenge free radicals, save your DNA, and leap tall buildings in a single bound.

Pyridoxamine is not one of these agents. It is understated, and really only does one thing; but sometimes all you need is one thing! Sometimes, you just need a specialist.

In order to cover all of the bases to prevent aging, one of the important pieces remaining is that of AGE products. There aren't that many things that prevent AGE production and accumulation, luckily, pyridoxamine is one of them.

• •

> *"Agents that have been found to affect tissue and/or circulating AGE levels include aspirin, thiamine, thiazolidinediones, carnosines, ACE inhibitors, ARBs (angiotensin receptor blockers), and Pyridoxamine."*[1]

• •

Pyridoxamine is part of the vitamin B6 family, together with pyridoxal and pyridoxine, but it is the only one that has the gift of AGE inhibition. It is also a benign substance; we already have a bit in our systems naturally.

If you recall from the chapter on Waste Management, the reaction of glucose and oxidative stress with proteins creates Advanced Glycation End products, or AGEs. These in turn, are responsible for innumerable, unfortunate cellular events. The other thing you may recall is that AGEs and the associated pathologies are responsible for many of the debilitating effects of diabetes. Thus, there has been a plethora of research looking into whether or not pyridoxamine can reduce any of the negative conditions associated with diabetes. The results are in, and of course it can!

● ●

> *"The discovery that pyridoxine (PM) can inhibit glycation reactions and the formation of advanced glycation end products (AGEs) stimulated new interest in this B6 vitamer as a prospective pharmacological agent for treatment of complications of diabetes."*[2]

> *"PM is a potent inhibitor of the formation of advanced glycation end products (AGEs), protein modifications that have been implicated in the pathogenesis of vascular complications of diabetes and aging."*[2]

● ●

The other thing to recall is that even normal amounts of glucose and fructose in our bodies eventually lead to the same complications that we see in diabetics, albeit a bit slower. Therefore, it makes sense that if we can block AGE production enough to help with diabetes, it will also slow down aging.

How exactly does pyridoxamine work? Some of this may sound familiar, but honestly, I'm including this only for the biochemists in the audience.

● ●

> *"The mechanism of action of PM includes: (i) inhibition of AGE formation by blocking oxidative degradation of the Amadori intermediate of the Maillard reaction; (ii) scavenging toxic carbonyl products of glucose and lipid degradation; and (iii) trapping of reactive oxygen species."*[2]

● ●

So, biochemically, it prevents the formation of AGE and ALE products. Meanwhile, in the body, it can protect many different organs. In fact, it can protect all of them.

Studies have shown that it can reduce kidney damage, reduce retinal damage and even reduce AGE accumulation in the skin of diabetic animals.

• •

> *"The results of animal studies suggest a link between PM inhibition of AGE formation and its therapeutic effects in diabetic complications. PM inhibited the progression of early renal disease, decreased hyperlipidemia and protect against a range of pathological changes in the retina of STZ-diabetic rats."[2]*

• •

Elevated blood pressure with aging and with diabetes is also linked to AGEs. In fact, the ability of AGEs to form the crosslinks on aortic collagen is one of the central underlying processes responsible for the increased arterial stiffening. By blocking the formation and thus the deposition of AGEs on collagen, the elasticity of vascular walls and thus normal blood pressure can be preserved. Conveniently, this also helps to protect your skin, as collagen resides there as well.

• •

> *"Prevention of the diabetes-related aortic stiffness by PM treatment parallels the reduction of AGE accumulation on collagen in the wall of the elastic reservoir."[3]*

> *"In diabetic rats, PM was shown to inhibit the progression of retinopathy and attenuated the accumulation of AGEs on aortic collagen."[4]*

• •

To drive home the message that pyridoxamine helps with diabetic complications, let's look at a really cool study of diabetic mice with back pain. First, they demonstrated that diabetes inflicts substantial damage on the spine; it destroys both the bone and the discs, leading to nerve compression and pain. The study added an anti-inflammatory medication, pentosanpolysulfate, and pyridoxine to the mouse diets. They discovered that blocking the inflammatory pathway in addition to limiting the creation of AGEs really benefitted the mice. Many of the debilitating and degenerative changes were reduced or prevented. [5]

After a few zillion studies in the literature touting the positive effects of pyridoxamine on diabetic complications, it became obvious a few years back that the agent was useful. Thus, it wasn't long until a drug company tried to turn it into a real medication. The company, Biostratum, started testing and producing a drug called Pyridorin, in which the active ingredient was pyridoxamine. The complicating factor here was that our B6 vitamin was already over the counter. Another complicating factor was money; the company cancelled the phase 3 trials in 2005 because they were out of cash. A battle then ensued between the FDA, the drug company and the supplement representatives.

Who won? We did (so far). At the moment, you can get pyridoxamine over the counter.

Is it safe? In human toxicity studies, it was found to be well tolerated and showed a favorable safety profile with no reported adverse effects. Human studies have also used varying doses, anywhere from 50 mg twice a day to 250 mg twice a day.

Kaufmann Number: 0.0.0.0.0.0.3

CHAPTER 25:

THE LAST CHAPTER

By now, you are well versed in the reasons that cause us to age. As more research is done, the list may become more extensive and undoubtedly it will become more specific; but for now, I told you all there is to know (with a few simplifications).

You have also become familiar with the top supplements and adjuvants that can ward off these evils. Therefore, rather than taking something because you 'heard it was good for you,' hopefully now you have enough information to make some educated decisions.

So, it is almost time to formulate a plan; but first, a few caveats.

1. This is not a diet book (I said this in the beginning, but it is important to reiterate). It isn't a 30 day, eat bacon and lose weight plan. It isn't a bowel cleanse. It isn't paleolithic. You may lose weight and you will definitely feel better, but that is not the primary goal.

2. This is not a fad. This is not designed as a short term fix. You will be aging your entire life, and it is a battle that will last for years. I am simply giving you the tools with which to design your own strategy.

3. You will feel better at first on this regime, and then you will level off. In the plateau period, you may not think anything substantial is happening and lose faith, but you need to remember that aging is constant. Therefore, even stagnation is success... because anything that decelerates the rate of deterioration is an absolute win.

4. You need to accept that we can't predict the future. There is no way of knowing if you are going to get cancer, diabetes, or any other disease of aging. The only thing we can actively do is decrease the relative risk of such things.

5. There aren't any studies presently demonstrating that these theories and treatments can actually elongate human life. In about a hundred years, there will be; but, as you well know, none of us will be here in a hundred years. Therefore, you can either wait and do nothing, or be proactive.

Now, the plan.

1. The first thing you need to do is take the aging questionnaire. It is important to establish a baseline prior to embarking on any plan. It will guide you into considering how you act and feel presently, and what aspects of aging are bothering you the most. As you begin to follow the protocol, you will change. Your energy levels will increase, your body will feel different and your life outlook will improve. I have discovered that without documenting a baseline, most people soon forget how they felt prior to initiating the protocol.

2. Decide what molecular agents you want to start with. You may have developed opinions while reading through all of the agents. For example, you may prefer natural versus man-made substances. You may like agents that have been around for centuries versus more recent discoveries. You may even choose certain agents by their secondary effects, such as weight loss or anti-inflammatory actions. Regardless, feel free to start with as many or as few as you desire.

If however, you want to go with my suggestions, I am happy to help. I usually offer a recommendation of what I consider the Top 5 agents.

Your Total **48**	TENET 1 DNA Alterations	TENET 2 Mitochondri-al Failure	TENET 3 Aging Pathways	TENET 4 Quality Control	TENET 5 Immune Sytem Failure	TENET 6 Individual Cell Needs	TENET 7 Waste Man-agement
Astaxanthin	0	3	0	0	2	0	0
Carnosine	0	3	0	0	0	0	3
Curcumin	2	3	1	0	3	0	3
Nicotinamide	0	3	3	3	0	0	0
Pterostilbene/ Resveratrol	2	3	3	3	2	2	1
	4	15	7	6	7	2	7

This brings you to a total score of: 4.15.7.6.2.7=48. All categories are covered, and you are off to a great start!

Some people following this program jump in and begin all five at the same time. Other folks are more cautious and prefer to try one at a time and slowly build up. Either strategy is valid. The important thing is that all aging categories are eventually covered.

3. Once you have decided on your agents, keep tract of them. Make sure you include the date you started as well as a few notes as you go along. Include both improvements and possible set backs.

In my experience, it takes ten to fourteen days to feel a difference. This is, of course, very dependent on the individual. Older people are going to take a little longer; active people tend to notice the difference faster. People with specific complaints tend to notice changes more readily as well. Regardless, the improvement is going to be subtle, but lasting. As well, there is no "high" feeling, only an improved feeling.

4. In two months, retake the aging questionnaire. You will undoubtedly feel different than you did before.

At this point you can either add a few agents, or even trade them out. Just remember that you need to follow the strategy of covering all of the bases.

On that note, I bid you farewell and good luck.

DOSES

RESVERATROL
100-250 mg/day up to
500 mg to 1 gm/day

PTEROSTILBENE
50 to 150 mg 2 times/day
Take with food

ASTAXANTHIN
2 to 12 mg (4-6 maintenance,
athletes 12 mg) Take with food

NICOTINAMIDE (RIBOSIDE)
250 to 500 mg /day

CURCUMIN
Dose depends on
particular formulation

CARNOSINE
500 mg 2 times/day
(Can't take at one time...
get skin paresthesias)

METFORMIN
500 to 2,000 mg/ day

ALPHA LIPOIC ACID
300-600 mg/day
(diabetic treatment
600 to 1,800 mg/day)
Do not take with food

APIGENIN
50 mg/day

SULFORAPHANE
Dose depends on
particular formulation

QUERCETIN
500 to 1,000 mg/day

EGCG
400-500 mg/day
one cup green tea = 50 mg
Take without food

ASTRAGALUS
TA-65: 100 to 250 units/day
Cycloastrogenol 5 to 25 mg/day
Astragaloside IV 50mg/day

MELATONIN
3 to 10 mg/ QD
Take at night

PYRIDOXAMINE
50 to 250 mg/day

ASSESSMENT & PROGRESS QUIZ

Why do I need to answer these questions?

I have learned over the many years of the protocol that people have very short term memories. Prior to initiating the therapy, people have very specific complaints about how they feel; aches and pains, infections, bad skin etc. After a month or so, however, when these complains dissipate, they seem to forget about them.

Thus, this questionnaire will serve two purposes. First, it will establish a baseline in certain health and aging categories.

Secondly, this exam needs to be repeated at monthly intervals. This will not only demonstrate real progress, but it will also bring to light additional aspects of aging that need to be addressed.

1. **WEIGHT:** _____ (lbs)

2. **PRESENT BLOOD PRESSURE:** _____

3. **RESTING HEART RATE:** _____

4. **MY OVERALL ENERGY LEVEL:**
   1 2 3 4 5 6 7 8 9 10
   (Terrible to Fantastic)

5. **MY PRESENT ACTIVITY LEVEL:**
   1 2 3 4 5 6 7 8 9 10
   (Not Active to Very Active)

6. **MY SEX DRIVE OR LIBIDO:**
   1 2 3 4 5 6 7 8 9 10
   (Terrible to Very Active)

7. **I FEEL EXHAUSTED BY MID DAY :**
1 2 3 4 5 6 7 8 9 10
(Wiped out to Endless Energy)

8. **I AM HAPPY WITH MY BODY SHAPE:**
1 2 3 4 5 6 7 8 9 10
(Not At All to I Look Amazing)

9. **I AM HAPPY WITH MY SKIN:**
1 2 3 4 5 6 7 8 9 10
(Not At All to It's Fantastic)

10. **I GET RESPIRATORY INFECTIONS:** (Colds, runny nose, pneumonia)
I am always sick **(1)**   Every month **(2)**   2-4 x year **(3)**   1 x year **(4)**   Never **(5)**

11. **I HAVE ALLERGIES:** (Pollen, dogs, etc.)
1 2 3 4 5 6 7 8 9 10
(Terrible to Not At All)

12. **MY PATTERN OF HAIR LOSS OR THINNING:**
1 2 3 4 5 6 7 8 9 10
(Significant Hair Loss to Not At All)

13. **I HAVE BACK PAIN, CHRONIC JOINT PAIN OR STIFFNESS:**
Always **(1)**   Daily **(2)**   Weekly **(3)**   After exercise only **(4)**   Never **(5)**

14. **PAIN LEVEL:**
1 2 3 4 5 6 7 8 9 10
(Absolute Misery to Very Little)

15. **I HAVE TROUBLE SLEEPING:**
1 2 3 4 5 6 7 8 9 10
(I Can't Sleep a Bit to I Sleep Very Well)

16. **MY DAYTIME VISION IS:**
1 2 3 4 5 6 7 8 9 10
(Terrible to Fantastic)

17. **MY NIGHT TIME VISION IS:**
1 2 3 4 5 6 7 8 9 10
(Terrible to Fantastic)

18. **MY UP CLOSE VISION IS:**
1 2 3 4 5 6 7 8 9 10
(Terrible to Fantastic)

19. **I RATE MY MEMORY AS:**
1 2 3 4 5 6 7 8 9 10
(I Can't Remember a Thing to Iron Clad Memory)

20. **I WOULD RATE MY DIET AS:**
1 2 3 4 5 6 7 8 9 10
(Terrible to Fantastic)

Summary:

WEIGHT: _____

BLOOD PRESSURE: _____

RESTING HEART RATE: _____

SCORE OUT OF 160: _____

PERCENTAGE: _____

GLOSSARY

Adaptive Immune System

A component of the immune system; it retains the memory of the enemy.

Adjuvant

A substance that you don't already have within you. It is a brand new, traceable substance.

AGEs

Advanced Glycation End Product(s). Formed when sugar, usually glucose or fructose, latches onto a molecule under oxidative, stressful conditions.

ALEs

Advanced Lipid oxidation End products. Formed when a sugar non-enzymatically attaches to a lipid.

Alpha Lipoic Acid

One of our adjuvants, aka Thioctic acid, acetate replacing factor, billet, lipoicin, or pyruvate oxidation factor. Scientifically, it is 1,2 - dithiolane-3-pentanoic acid.
Kaufmann Rating: 2.3.1.0.2.2.1

Aminoguanine

Recognized in 1986 as the first agent proposed to help in the eradication of AGEs. Not used today secondary side effects.

AMP

Adenosine monophosphate, a molecule having a lower state of energy than ATP.

AMP Kinase

Adenosine Monophosphate-activated Protein Kinase. A central regulator of cellular and organismal metabolism that plays a critical role in maintaining energy homeostasis. Also known as the Metabolic Master Switch.

Anabolic Systems

Processes that build things.

Antibodies

Y shaped proteins that come in a variety of configurations (different numbers of Y's stuck together). They identify and adhere to specific pathogens.

Antioxidant

A molecule that inhibits the oxidation of other molecules. Oxidation is a chemical reaction that can produce free radicals, leading to chain reactions that may damage cells.

Apigenin

One of our adjuvants, also one of the main active substances in Chamomile tea.
Kaufmann Rating: 2.1.0.1.2.0.0

Apoptosis

Programmed cell death.

Astaxanthin

One of our supplements, a xanthophyll carotenoid.
Kaufmann Rating: 0.3.0.0.2.0.0

Astragalus Radix Membranaceus
Used in Chinese medicine for over 2,000 years and strengthens the "Qi". Composed of cycloastrogenol, astragaloside IV and innumerable other components.
Kaufmann Rating: 3.0.0.0.2.1.0

ATP
Adenosine Tri-Phosphate. The cellular or molecular unit of energy currency.

Autophagy
Literally means "eating oneself." A catabolic pathway that promotes the degradation and recycling of cellular components.

Base Excision Repair (BER)
The most basic DNA repair system, deals with single lesions or small alterations of bases. Usually repairs single strand problems.

Blood Brain Barrier
A real barrier that separates blood flow from brain tissue as it flows through the cranium. The barrier functions to keep toxins and unwanted molecules out of the brain.

BMAL1
Brain and muscle-ARNT-like 1. Part of the daytime functioning protein family. Controls circadian rhythms.

Caloric Restriction
A 30% (sometime 20 to 50%) reduction in calories without starvation from a standard diet

Caloric Restriction Mimetics
Metformin, Resveratrol, Pterostilbene, EGCG, Quercetin, Curcumin

Carnosine
A naturally occurring dipeptide, made of L-histidine and B-alanine.
Kaufmann Rating: 0.3.0.0.0.0.3

Catabolic Mechanisms
Processes that break things into smaller pieces.

Catalase
A common enzyme found in nearly all living organisms exposed to oxygen. It catalyzes the decomposition of hydrogen peroxide to water and oxygen.

Cell Cycle arrest
When a cell stays in the same stage of life.

Cellular Proteome
The entire pool of cellular protein.

Chamomile Tea
The major source of apigenin. Other compounds include alpha-bisabolol, quercetin and 120 secondary metabolites, including 28 terpenoids and 36 flavonoids.

Chaparones

Proteins that accompany other
larger proteins throughout their
proteinaceous lives. The chaperones
duty is to protect the protein as it
morphs into different shapes and
guard it from attack when it
is vulnerable.

Codon

A triplet of base pairs in the DNA,
codes for each of the 20 amino acids
found in humans.

Collagen

Molecules that provide the structural
framework in most organs, can stretch
about 10%.

CLOCK

The Circadian Locomotor Output
Cycles Kaput. Located mainly in
the suprachiasmatic nucleus of
the hypothalamus.

Curcumin

The active substance from
the spice turmeric.
Kaufmann Rating: 2.3.1.0.3.0.3

Dentate Gyrus

An area in the brain, specifically in
the hippocampus. It contributes to the
formation of new, episodic memories
and the spontaneous exploration of
novel environments.

Cyclobutane Pyrimidine Dimers

CPD's. Complexes that form when the
DNA is "melted" together.

Diabetes

A disease of hyperglycemia.
Type I diabetes is an autoimmune
disease, usually effecting younger
people.The body makes antibodies
that attacks the pancreas such that
insulin cannot be produced normally.
Type II diabetes is much more
prevalent, and is associated with
being overweight, aging and having
a poor diet.

DNA

Deoxyribonucleic acid.
Base pairs are Adenine, Thymine,
Guanine and Cytosine

DNA Damage

Measured by 8-hydroxy-2-
deoxyguanosine

DNA Damage Response System

DDR, A system with four main
components: damage sensors,
signal transducers, repair effectors,
and cell arrest.

DNA Methyltransferase

DNMT. An enzyme that alters the
epigenetics of DNA, specifically
transferring a methyl group.

Epigallocatechin Gallate
EGCG. The most active ingredient in green tea. *Kaufmann Rating: 2.2.1.2.1.1.2.*

Epigenetics
The science of genetics beyond that of the base pair arrangement.

Epigenetic Clock
A method of determining age by examining specific sites of DNA methylation.

Epigenetic Diet
The consumption of certain foods, such as soy, grapes, cruciferous vegetables and green tea, which have been shown to induce epigenetic mechanisms that protect against cancer and aging.

Epigenetic Drift
Age-related changes in the epigenome that include those acquired both environmentally and stochastically.

Electron Transport Chain
A series of proteins embedded in the inner membrane of the mitochondria that create a chemical gradient in order to produce ATP.

Endosymbiosis Theory
A theory that mitochondrial were once independent cells that were engulfed into larger cells and now serve as their power supply.

Endoplasmic Reticulum
An organelle that is long and tubular and serves as an assembly line for protein production.

Free Radicals
An uncharged molecule or atom that has a single unpaired electron or any species capable of independent existence that contains one or more unpaired electrons. Examples include $O2^-$ (superoxide), HO (hydroxyl radical), O^- (oxygen singlet), $H2O2$ (hydrogen peroxide), and $ONOO^-$ (peroxynitrite).

Free Radical Scavenger
A molecule that is able to destroy free radicals.

Genotype
The traits that are coded for in the genes.

Glycation
The process of a sugar bonding with a second type of molecule.

Gluconeogenesis
The creation of new glucose molecules.

Hematopoiesis
The generation of blood cells.

Hippocampus
A bilateral area in the brain associated with memory formation.

Histamine

A molecule responsible for dilating blood vessels, and recruiting inflammatory factors, and causing pruritus.

Histone Deacetylase

HDAC. An enzyme that alters the epigenetics of DNA, specifically removing an acetyl group.

Hydralazine

A medication generally used to treat high blood pressure that can actually prevent AGE formation.

Innate immune system

The first line of immune defense.

Killer T Cells

Immune cells that find and destroy infected human cells that have been compromised.

Leukocytes

White blood cells. There are innumerable types of white cells, but the most important are the neutrophils and the macrophages.

Lipolysis

The breakdown of fat and triglycerides.

Lipofuscin

An intracellular, indigestible material mainly composed of oxidized proteins and lipids.

Macrophages

A subtype of white blood cells. (i.e. Big Eaters, by Greek roots) They congregate several days after an initiating event, and replace the neutrophils as the predominant cell type.

Mast Cells

A less numerous subtype of white blood cells. They play a role in wound healing, blood vessels production (angiogenesis), and protection of the blood-brain barrier. Importantly, these cells release histamine.

Melatonin

An ancient molecule, technically an endogenously produced indolamine. *Kaufmann Rating: 2.2.1.2.2.2.0*

Metformin

A prescription medication known by the trade name Glucophage. Used for the control of diabetes. *Kaufmann Rating: 3.1.3.2.2.2.3*

Mitochondria

Intracellular organelles that specialize in energy production.

Mitosis

cell division whereby the contents of each daughter cell is identical.

MTOR

A pathway that is essential for growth and development when you are young.

Nicotinamide
One of the key supplements.
Necessary for energy production,
DNA repair, sirtuins, and
cellular communication.
Kaufmann Rating: 0.3.3.3.0.0.0

Neutrophils
The most common type of white blood
cell, they constitute about 60 to 70% of
the circulating white blood cells.

Nuclear Factor (erythroid-derived 2) like 2 (Nrf2)
A transcription factor that activates a
series of endogenous anti-oxidants.
These include heme-oxygenate-1,
glutamate cysteine ligase, glutathione
Stransferase, glutathione peroxidase,
superoxide dismutase, catalase,
sulfiredoxin and thioredoxin.

Nuclear Factor Kappa-Beta
A cytokine at the apex of the
inflammatory cascade.

Nucleotide Excision Repair
NER. A process of DNA repair
which excises bigger or bulky pieces
of the DNA.

Osteoblasts
Bone cells that build new bone.

Osteoclasts
Bone cells that work demolition.

Oxidation
Loss of an electron, an increase in the
oxidative state.

Pancreas
An important abdominal organ that
produces insulin.

Pathogens
Any biological agent that can harm or
bring disease to its host.

Period 1
PERs. A night time protein family,
associated with CRYs (Cryptochrome
1 and 2).

Phenotype
What traits get seen in an individual.

Phytoalexin
A substance produced by plants when
said plant gets stressed out.

Poly-ADP-Ribose Polymerase
PARPs. An enzyme that senses and
repairs breaks in DNA.

Proteostasis
The homeostasis of protein
production, it is the ability of a cell to
synthesize, fold and turnover proteins.

Proteotoxicity
Maladapted proteins that become toxic.

Protons

H+ atoms

Pterostilbene

A stillbene related to resveratrol.
Mostly derived from blueberries.
Kaufmann Rating: 2.3.3.3.2.2.1

Pyridoxamine

A subtype of vitamin B6 and a
recommended supplement.
Kaufmann Rating: 0.0.0.0.0.0.3

Pyrimidine Pyrimidones

A molecular complex that forms when
the DNA is "melted together".

Quercetin

A ubiquitous flavenoid.
Kaufmann Rating: 0.3.1.2.2.2.0

Rapamycin

A medication that is used for its
immunosuppressant qualities. It is
also the key substance that identified
the mTOR pathway.

Reductive

The gain of an electron or decrease in
oxidative state.

Resveratrol

A stilbene found in many foods
including red wine.
Kaufmann Rating: 2.3.3.3.2.2.1

Senescence

A type of retirement for cells. Rather
than dying, they remain active but end
up harming the organism.

**Senescence-Associated
Secretory Phenotype**

SASP. The production and release
of degradative enzymes, proteases
and inflammatory cytokines as well
as other compounds that negatively
effect the environment of the cell.

Sirtuins

Silent Information Regulator gene
famil. A family of genes that regulates
the bodies metabolic and growth
pathways. They sense the environment
in terms of energy availability, timing
of daylight, environmental stressors
and alters the metabolism to promote
survival.

Stem Cells

undifferentiated, long-lived cells that
are unique in their abilities to produce
differentiated daughter cells and to
retain their stem cell identity by
self-renewal.

Sulforaphane

An isothiocyanate molecule found
in cruciferous vegetables, especially
in broccoli, but it is also in kale,
cabbage, and brussel sprouts.
Kaufmann Rating: 3.2.0.1.0.2.0

Supplement

An agent that you can take that you already actually have in your body. You are simply adding to the total quantity.

Superoxide Dismutase

Endogenous enzymes that scavenge free radicals. Copper/Zinc Superoxide Dismutase (SOD1), Manganese Superoxide Dismutase (MnSOD or SOD2), SOD3 (Copper/ Zinc)

Telomeres

The ends of DNA. The length of which correlates with the expected length of life.

Telomerase

An endogenous enzyme that creates longer telomeres.

Telomerase Reverse Transcriptase

TERT. An endogenous enzyme that creates longer telomeres.

Tumor necrosis Factor (TNF)

An inflammatory cytokine that sits at the top of the inflammatory cascade.

Ubiquitin/Proteasome System

UPS. The major cellular system for selective removal of misfiled or damaged proteins

UVA Radiation

(wavelength 320-400 nm) Constitutes much more of the solar radiation that reaches us, about 90 to 95%. Known as the "aging ray".

UVB

(wavelengths of between 280-320 nm) Represents about 5% of solar radiation and penetrates the entire epidermis and into the dermis.

	DNA Alterations	Mito-chondria	Aging Pathways	Quality Control	The Security System	Individual Cell Needs	Waste Management	Total Points
Alpha Lipoic Acid	2	3	1	0	2	2	1	11
Apigenin	2	1	0	1	2	0	0	6
Astaxanthin	0	3	0	0	2	0	0	5
Astragalus	3	0	0	0	2	1	0	6
Carnosine	0	3	0	0	0	0	3	6
Curcumin	2	3	1	0	3	0	3	12
EGCG	2	2	1	2	1	1	2	11

Melatonin	2	2	1	2	2	2	0	11
Metformin	3	1	3	2	2	2	3	16
Nicotinamide Riboside	0	3	3	3	0	0	0	9
Pyridoxamine	0	0	0	0	0	0	3	3
Quercetin	0	3	1	2	2	2	0	10
Resveratrol/Ptero	2	3	3	3	2	2	1	16
Sulforaphane	3	2	0	1	0	2	0	8

CITATIONS

INTRODUCTION

1. Barbieri, Elena, et al. "The pleiotropic effect of physical exercise on mitochondrial dynamics in aging skeletal muscle." *Oxidative medicine and cellular longevity* 2015 (2015).

2. Barzilai, Nir, et al. "The critical role of metabolic pathways in aging." *Diabetes* 61.6 (2012): 1315-1322.

3. Carmona, Juan José, and Shaday Michan. "Biology of healthy aging and longevity." *Rev Invest Clin* 68.1 (2016): 7-16.

GENETIC CONTROL

1. Bormann, Felix, et al. "Reduced DNA methylation patterning and transcriptional connectivity define human skin aging." *Aging cell* 15.3 (2016): 563-571.

2. Daniel, Michael, and Trygve O. Tollefsbol. "Epigenetic linkage of aging, cancer and nutrition." *Journal of Experimental Biology* 218.1 (2015): 59-70.

3. Horvath, Steve. "DNA methylation age of human tissues and cell types." *Genome biology* 14.10 (2013): 3 56.

4. Jones, Meaghan J., Sarah J. Goodman, and Michael S. Kobor. "DNA methylation and healthy human aging." *Aging cell* 14.6 (2015): 924-932.

5. Issa, Jean-Pierre. "Aging and epigenetic drift: a vicious cycle." *The Journal of clinical investigation* 124.1 (2014): 24-29.

6. Remely, M., et al. "Therapeutic perspectives of epigenetically active nutrients." *British journal of pharmacology* 172.11 (2015): 2756-2768.

MITOCHONDRIA

1. Whatley, Jean M., P. John, and F. R. Whatley. "From extracellular to intracellular: the establishment of mitochondria and chloroplasts." *Proceedings of the Royal Society of London B: Biological Sciences* 204.1155 (1979): 165-187.

2. Stuart, Jeffrey A., et al. "A midlife crisis for the mitochondrial free radical theory of aging." *Longevity & healthspan* 3.1 (2014): 4.

3. Tilly, Jonathan L., and David A. Sinclair. "Germline energetics, aging, and female infertility." *Cell metabolism* 17.6 (2013): 838-850.

4. Bentov, Yaakov, et al. "The contribution of mitochondrial function to reproductive aging." *Journal of assisted reproduction and genetics* 28.9 (2011): 773-783.

5. Ziegler, Dorian V., Christopher D. Wiley, and Michael C. Velarde. "Mitochondrial effectors of cellular senescence: beyond the free radical theory of aging." *Aging cell* 14.1 (2015): 1-7.

6. Indo, Hiroko P., et al. "A mitochondrial superoxide theory for oxidative stress diseases and aging." *Journal of clinical biochemistry and nutrition* 56.1 (2015): 1-7.

7. Wood, John M., et al. "Senile hair graying: H2O2-mediated oxidative stress affects human hair color by blunting methionine sulfoxide repair." *The FASEB Journal* 23.7 (2009): 2065-2075.

8. Cantó, Carles, and Johan Auwerx. "Interference between PARPs and SIRT1: a novel approach to healthy ageing?." *Aging (Albany NY)* 3.5 (2011): 543-547.

9. Stein, Liana Roberts, and Shin-ichiro Imai. "The dynamic regulation of NAD metabolism in mitochondria." *Trends in Endocrinology & Metabolism* 23.9 (2012): 420-428.

10. Gomes, Ana P., et al. "Declining NAD+ induces a pseudohypoxic state disrupting nuclear-mitochondrial communication during aging." *Cell* 155.7 (2013): 1624-1638.

PATHWAYS

Section Caloric Restriction/AMP Kinase

1. Willcox, D. Craig, et al. "Caloric restriction and human longevity: what can we learn from the Okinawans?." *Biogerontology* 7.3 (2006): 173-177.

2. Testa, Gabriella, et al. "Calorie restriction and dietary restriction mimetics: a strategy for improving healthy aging and longevity." *Current pharmaceutical design*

20.18 (2014): 2950-2977.

3. Li, Yuanyuan, Michael Daniel, and Trygve O. Tollefsbol. "Epigenetic regulation of caloric restriction in aging." *BMC medicine* 9.1 (2011): 98.

4. Sohal, Rajindar S., and Michael J. Forster. "Caloric restriction and the aging process: a critique." *Free Radical Biology and Medicine* 73 (2014): 366-382.

5. Salminen, Antero, Juha MT Hyttinen, and Kai Kaarniranta. "AMP-activated protein kinase inhibits NF-κB signaling and inflammation: impact on healthspan and lifespan." *Journal of molecular medicine* 89.7 (2011): 667-676.

6. Salminen, Antero, and Kai Kaarniranta. "AMP-activated protein kinase (AMPK) controls the aging process via an integrated signaling network." *Ageing research reviews* 11.2 (2012): 230-241.

Sirtuin Section

7. Salminen, Antero, Kai Kaarniranta, and Anu Kauppinen. "Crosstalk between oxidative stress and SIRT1: impact on the aging process." *International journal of molecular sciences* 14.2 (2013): 3834-3859.

8. Covington, Jeffrey D., and Sudip Bajpeyi. "The sirtuins: markers of metabolic health." *Molecular nutrition & food research* 60.1 (2016): 79-91.

9. Masri, Selma. "Sirtuin-dependent clock control: new advances in metabolism, aging and cancer." *Current opinion in clinical nutrition and metabolic care* 18.6 (2015): 521-527.

10. Hall, Jessica A., et al. "The sirtuin family's role in aging and age-associated pathologies." *The Journal of clinical investigation* 123.3 (2013): 973-979.

11. Brown, Katharine, et al. "SIRT3 reverses aging-associated degeneration." *Cell reports* 3.2 (2013): 319-327.

mTOR Section

12. Lamming, Dudley W., et al. "Rapalogs and mTOR inhibitors as anti-aging·therapeutics." *The Journal of clinical investigation* 123.3 (2013): 980-989.

13. Laplante, Mathieu, and David M. Sabatini. "mTOR signaling at a glance." *Journal of cell science* 122.20 (2009): 3589-3594.

14. Blagosklonny, Mikhail V. "Rapamycin extends life-and health span because it slows aging." *Aging* (Albany NY) 5.8 (2013): 592-598.

15. Johnson, Simon C., Peter S. Rabinovitch, and Matt Kaeberlein. "mTOR is a key modulator of ageing and age-related disease." *Nature* 493.7432 (2013): 338-345.

16. Bitto, Alessandro, et al. "Transient rapamycin treatment can increase lifespan and healthspan in middle-aged mice." *Elife* 5 (2016): e16351.

17. Wilkinson, John E., et al. "Rapamycin slows aging in mice." *Aging cell* 11.4 (2012): 675-682.

MAINTENANCE DEPARTMENT

1. Moehrle, Bettina M., and Hartmut Geiger. "Aging of hematopoietic stem cells: DNA damage and mutations?." *Experimental*

Hematology 44.10 (2016): 895-901.

2. Panich, Uraiwan, et al. "Ultraviolet radiation-induced skin aging: the role of DNA damage and oxidative stress in epidermal stem cell damage mediated skin aging." *Stem cells international* 2016 (2016).

3. Ermolaeva, Maria A., Alexander Dakhovnik, and Björn Schumacher. "Quality control mechanisms in cellular and systemic DNA damage responses." *Ageing research reviews* 23 (2015): 3-11.

4, Nichols, Joi A., and Santosh K. Katiyar. "Skin photoprotection by natural polyphenols: anti-inflammatory, antioxidant and DNA repair mechanisms." *Archives of dermatological research* 302.2 (2010): 71-83.

5. Koga, Hiroshi, Susmita Kaushik, and Ana Maria Cuervo. "Protein homeostasis and aging: The importance of exquisite quality control." *Ageing research reviews* 10.2 (2011): 205-215.

6. Sontag, Emily M., Willianne IM Vonk, and Judith Frydman. "Sorting out the trash: the spatial nature of eukaryotic protein quality control." *Current opinion in cell biology* 26 (2014): 139-146.

7. Ziv, Ilan, and Eldad Melamed. "Editorial: apoptosis in the aging brain." *Apoptosis* 15.11 (2010): 1285-1291.

8. Riederer, Beat M., et al. "The role of the ubiquitin proteasome system in Alzheimer's disease." *Experimental Biology and Medicine* 236.3 (2011): 268-276.

9. Martinez-Lopez, Nuria, Diana

Athonvarangkul, and Rajat Singh. "Autophagy and aging." _Longevity Genes._ Springer New York, 2015. 73-87.

10. Ikeda, Yoshiyuki, et al. "New insights into the role of mitochondrial dynamics and autophagy during oxidative stress and aging in the heart." _Oxidative medicine and cellular longevity_ 2014 (2014).

SECURITY

1. vel Szic, Katarzyna Szarc, et al. "From inflammaging to healthy aging by dietary lifestyle choices: is epigenetics the key to personalized nutrition?." _Clinical epigenetics_ 7.1 (2015): 33.

2. Adriaensen, Dirk, Inge Brouns, and Jean-Pierre Timmermans. "Sensory input to the central nervous system from the lungs and airways: A prominent role for purinergic signalling via P2X2/3 receptors." _Autonomic Neuroscience_ 191 (2015): 39-47.

3. Franceschi, Claudio, and Judith Campisi. "Chronic inflammation (inflammaging) and its potential contribution to ageassociated diseases." _The Journals of Gerontology Series A: Biological Sciences and Medical Sciences_ 69.Suppl 1 (2014): S4-S9.

4. de Mora, Jaime Font, and Antonio Díez Juan. "The decay of stem cell nourishment at the niche." _Rejuvenation research_ 16.6 (2013): 487-494.

5. Jurenka, J. S. "Anti-inflammatory Properties of Curcumin, a Major Constituent of Curcuma Longa: A Review of Preclinical and Clinical Research (vol 14, pg 141, 2009)." _Alternative Medicine Review_ 14.3 (2009): 277-277.

6. Hawkes, Jason E., and Ryan M. O'Connell. "MicroRNAs, T follicular helper cells and inflammaging." _Oncotarget_ 6.32 (2015): 32295.

CELL CHALLENGES

1. Spalding, Kirsty L., et al. "Dynamics of hippocampal neurogenesis in adult humans." _Cell_ 153.6 (2013): 1219-1227.

2. Ziv, Ilan, and Eldad Melamed. "Editorial: apoptosis in the aging brain." _Apoptosis_ 15.11 (2010): 1285-1291.

3. Almeida, Maria, and Charles A. O'Brien. "Basic biology of skeletal aging: role of stress response pathways." _The Journals of Gerontology Series A: Biological Sciences and Medical Sciences_ (2013): glt079.

4. Spalding, Kirsty L., et al. "Dynamics of fat cell turnover in humans." _Nature_ 453.7196 (2008): 783-787.

5. Cnop, Miriam, et al. "Longevity of human islet α-and β-cells." _Diabetes, obesity and metabolism_ 13.s1 (2011): 39-46.

6. Cheung, Tom H., and Thomas A. Rando. "Molecular regulation of stem cell quiescence." Nature reviews _Molecular cell biology_ 14.6 (2013): 329-340.

7. Wiley, Christopher, and Judith Campisi. "NAD+ controls neural

stem cell fate in the aging brain." *The EMBO journal* 33.12 (2014): 1289-1291.

8. Lay, Kenneth, Tsutomu Kume, and Elaine Fuchs. "FOXC1 maintains the hair follicle stem cell niche and governs stem cell quiescence to preserve long-term tissue-regenerating potential." *Proceedings of the National Academy of Sciences* (2016): 201601569.

9. Shin, Jiyung, Mary Mohrin, and Danica Chen. "Reversing stem cell aging." (2015): 14723-14724.

10. Geiger, Hartmut, Gerald De Haan, and M. Carolina Florian. "The ageing haematopoietic stem cell compartment." *Nature Reviews Immunology* 13.5 (2013): 376-389.

11. Oh, Juhyun, Yang David Lee, and Amy J. Wagers. "Stem cell aging: mechanisms, regulators and therapeutic opportunities." *Nature medicine* 20.8 (2014): 870-880.

12. Alt, Eckhard U., et al. "Aging alters tissue resident mesenchymal stem cell properties." *Stem cell research* 8.2 (2012): 215-225.

13. Adams, Peter D., Heinrich Jasper, and K. Lenhard Rudolph. "Aging-induced stem cell mutations as drivers for disease and cancer." *Cell stem cell* 16.6 (2015): 601-612.

14. Deng, W., et al. "Telomerase activity and its association with psychological stress, mental disorders, lifestyle factors and interventions: A systematic review." *Psychoneuroendocrinology* 64 (2016): 150-163.

15. Bouchard, Jill, and Saul A. Villeda. "Aging and brain rejuvenation as systemic events." Journal of neurochemistry 132.1 (2015): 5-19.

16. Panish, U. et al. "Ultraviolet Radiation-Induced Skin Aging: The Role of DNA Damage and Oxidative Stress in Epidermal Stem Cell Damage Mediated Skin Aging. Stem Cells International. 2016. Art ID# 7370642.

17. Oshima, Motohiko, and Atsushi Iwama. "Epigenetics of hematopoietic stem cell aging and disease." *International journal of hematology* 100.4 (2014): 326-334.

18. Wahlestedt, Martin, Cornelis Jan Pronk, and David Bryder. "Concise review: hematopoietic stem cell aging and the prospects for rejuvenation." *Stem cells translational medicine* 4.2 (2015): 186-194.

19. Childs, Bennett G., et al. "Senescence and apoptosis: dueling or complementary cell fates?." *EMBO reports* 15.11 (2014): 1139-1153.

WASTE MANAGEMENT

1. Ahmad, Saheem, et al. "Glycoxidation of biological macromolecules: A critical approach to halt the menace of glycation." *Glycobiology* (2014): cwu057.

2. Van Puyvelde, Katrien, et al. "Effect of advanced glycation end product intake on inflammation and aging: a systematic review." *Nutrition reviews* 72.10 (2014): 638-650.

3. Stirban, Alin, et al. "Acute macrovascular dysfunction in patients with type 2 diabetes induced by ingestion of advanced glycated β-lactoglobulins." *Diabetes*

care 36.5 (2013): 1278-1282.

4. Vistoli, G., et al. "Advanced
    glycoxidation and lipoxidation end
    products (AGEs and ALEs): an
    overview of their mechanisms of
    formation." _Free radical research_
    47.sup1 (2013): 3-27.

5. Sell, David R., and Vincent
    M. Monnier. "Molecular basis
    of arterial stiffening: role of
    glycation–a mini-review."
    Gerontology 58.3 (2012): 227-237.

6. Kesavan, Suresh K., et al.
    "Proteome wide reduction
    in AGE modification in
    streptozotocin induced diabetic
    mice by hydralazine mediated
    transglycation." _Scientific reports_ 3
    (2013): 2941.

7. Ahmad, Saheem, et al. "Inhibitory
    effect of metformin and
    pyridoxamine in the formation of
    early, intermediate and advanced
    glycation end-products." _PloS one_
    8.9 (2013): e72128.

8. Aldini, Giancarlo, et al. "Molecular
    strategies to prevent, inhibit, and
    degrade advanced glycoxidation
    and advanced lipoxidation end
    products." _Free radical research_
    47.sup1 (2013): 93-137.

Lipofuscin

9. Terman, Alexei. "Catabolic
    insufficiency and aging." _Annals of
    the New York Academy of Sciences_
    1067.1 (2006): 27-36.

10. Bayati, Samaneh, and Razieh
    Yazdanparast. "Antioxidant and
    free radical scavenging potential
    of yakuchinone B derivatives in
    reduction of lipofuscin formation
    using H2O2-treated neuroblastoma

cells." _Iranian biomedical journal_
    15.4 (2011): 134-142.

11. Kumar, Pardeep, et al. "Effect of
    dehydroepiandrosterone (DHEA)
    on monoamine oxidase activity,
    lipid peroxidation and lipofuscin
    accumulation in aging rat brain
    regions." _Biogerontology_ 9.4
    (2008): 235-246.

12. Maxwell, Kerry E., et al.
    "Neurolipofuscin is a measure
    of age in Panulirus argus, the
    Caribbean spiny lobster, in Florida."
    The Biological Bulletin 213.1
    (2007): 55-66.

13. Jung, Tobias, Nicolle Bader, and
    Tilman Grune. "Lipofuscin." Annals
    of the New York Academy of
    Sciences 1119.1 (2007): 97-111.

14. Bala, Kiran, B. C. Tripathy, and
    Deepak Sharma. "Neuroprotective
    and anti-ageing effects of curcumin
    in aged rat brain regions."
    Biogerontology 7.2 (2006): 81-89.

15. Cnop, Miriam, et al. "The long
    lifespan and low turnover of
    human islet beta cells estimated
    by mathematical modelling
    of lipofuscin accumulation."
    Diabetologia 53.2 (2010): 321.

RESVERATROL

1. Weiskirchen, Sabine, and Ralf
    Weiskirchen. "Resveratrol: how
    much wine do you have to drink
    to stay healthy?." _Advances in
    Nutrition: An International Review
    Journal_ 7.4 (2016): 706-718.

2. Tellone, Ester, et al. "Resveratrol: a
    focus on several neurodegenerative
    diseases." _Oxidative medicine and
    cellular longevity_ 2015 (2015).

3. Britton, Robert G., Christina Kovoor, and Karen Brown. "Direct molecular targets of resveratrol: identifying key interactions to unlock complex mechanisms." *Annals of the New York Academy of Sciences* 1348.1 (2015): 124-133.

4. Huang, Peixin, et al. "A critical role of nicotinamide phosphoribosyltransferase in human telomerase reverse transcriptase induction by resveratrol in aortic smooth muscle cells." *Oncotarget* 6.13 (2015): 10812.

5. Malhotra, Ashim, Sundeep Bath, and Fawzy Elbarbry. "An organ system approach to explore the antioxidative, anti-inflammatory, and cytoprotective actions of resveratrol." *Oxidative medicine and cellular longevity* 2015 (2015).

6. Villalba, José M., and Francisco J. Alcaín. "Sirtuin activators and inhibitors." *Biofactors* 38.5 (2012): 349-359.

7. Latruffe, Norbert, et al. "Exploring new ways of regulation by resveratrol involving miRNAs, with emphasis on inflammation." *Annals of the New York Academy of Sciences* 1348.1 (2015): 97-106.

8. Taguchi, Ayumi, et al. "Resveratrol suppresses inflammatory responses in endometrial stromal cells derived from endometriosis: a possible role of the sirtuin 1 pathway." Journal of Obstetrics and Gynaecology Research 40.3 (2014): 770-778.

9. Gambini, J., et al. "Properties of resveratrol: in vitro and in vivo studies about metabolism, bioavailability, and biological effects in animal models and humans." *Oxidative medicine and cellular longevity* 2015 (2015).

10. Lançon, Allan, Raffaele Frazzi, and Norbert Latruffe. "Anti-oxidant, anti-inflammatory and anti-angiogenic properties of resveratrol in ocular diseases." *Molecules* 21.3 (2016): 304.

11. Zhang, Q. B., et al. "Effects of Sirtuin 1 on the proliferation and osteoblastic differentiation of periodontal ligament stem cells and stem cells from apical papilla." *Genet Mol Res* 15 (2016).

12. Bruckbauer, Antje, and Michael B. Zemel. "Synergistic effects of metformin, resveratrol, and hydroxymethylbutyrate on insulin sensitivity." *Diabetes Metab Syndr Obes* 6 (2013): 93-102.

13. Monserrat Hernández-Hernández, Elizabeth, et al. "Chronic administration of resveratrol prevents morphological changes in prefrontal cortex and hippocampus of aged rats." *Synapse* (2016).

14. Witte, A. Veronica, et al. "Effects of resveratrol on memory performance, hippocampal functional connectivity, and glucose metabolism in healthy older adults." *Journal of Neuroscience* 34.23 (2014): 7862-7870.

15. Baile, Clifton A., et al. "Effect of resveratrol on fat mobilization." *Annals of the New York Academy of Sciences* 1215.1 (2011): 40-47.

16. Ortega, Israel, and Antoni J. Duleba. "Ovarian actions of resveratrol." *Annals of the New York Academy of Sciences* 1348.1 (2015): 86-96.

17. Tomé-Carneiro, Joao, et al.

"Resveratrol and clinical trials: the crossroad from in vitro studies to human evidence." *Current pharmaceutical design* 19.34 (2013): 6064-6093.

18. Chachay, Veronique S., et al. "Resveratrol–pills to replace a healthy diet?." *British journal of clinical pharmacology* 72.1 (2011): 27-38.

19. Stipp,D. Blog on Scientific American. "Beyond Resveratrol:The Anti-aging NAD fad. March 2015.

20. McFadden, David. "A review of pterostilbene antioxidant activity and disease modification." *Oxidative medicine and cellular longevity* 2013 (2013).

21. Kapetanovic, Izet M., et al. "Pharmacokinetics, oral bioavailability, and metabolic profile of resveratrol and its dimethylether analog, pterostilbene, in rats." *Cancer chemotherapy and pharmacology* 68.3 (2011): 593-601.

22. Riche, Daniel M., et al. "Analysis of safety from a human clinical trial with pterostilbene." *Journal of toxicology* 2013 (2013).

23. Joseph, James A., et al. "Cellular and behavioral effects of stilbene resveratrol analogues: implications for reducing the deleterious effects of aging." *Journal of agricultural and food chemistry* 56.22 (2008): 10544-10551.

24. Estrela, José M., et al. "Pterostilbene: biomedical applications." *Critical reviews in clinical laboratory sciences* 50.3 (2013): 65-78.

25. Acharya, Jhankar D., and Saroj S. Ghaskadbi. "Protective effect of Pterostilbene against free radical mediated oxidative damage." *BMC complementary and alternative medicine* 13.1 (2013): 238.

ASTAXANTHIN

1. Shah, Md Mahfuzur R., et al. "Astaxanthin-producing green microalga Haematococcus pluvialis: from single cell to high value commercial products." *Frontiers in plant science* 7 (2016).

2. Ambati, Ranga Rao, et al. "Astaxanthin: sources, extraction, stability, biological activities and its commercial applications—a review." *Marine drugs* 12.1 (2014): 128-152.

3. Zhang, Li, and Handong Wang. "Multiple mechanisms of anti-cancer effects exerted by astaxanthin." *Marine drugs* 13.7 (2015): 4310-4330.

4. Belviranli, Muaz, and Nilsel Okudan. "Well-Known Antioxidants and Newcomers in Sport Nutrition." (2015).

5. Park, Jean Soon, et al. "Astaxanthin decreased oxidative stress and inflammation and enhanced immune response in humans." *Nutrition & metabolism* 7.1 (2010): 18.

6. Yeh, Po-Ting, et al. "Astaxanthin inhibits expression of retinal oxidative stress and inflammatory mediators in streptozotocin-induced diabetic rats." *PloS one* 11.1 (2016): e0146438.

7. Wu, Haijian, et al. "Astaxanthin as a potential neuroprotective agent for neurological diseases." *Marine*

drugs 13.9 (2015): 5750-5766.

8. Kidd, Parris. "Astaxanthin, cell membrane nutrient with diverse clinical benefits and anti-aging potential." *Altern Med Rev* 16.4 (2011): 355-64.

9. Speranza, Lorenza, et al. "Astaxanthin treatment reduced oxidative induced pro-inflammatory cytokines secretion in U937: SHP-1 as a novel biological target." *Marine drugs* 10.4 (2012): 890-899.

10. Kim, Yeon Hyang, Hyung-Kon Koh, and Doo-Sik Kim. "Down-regulation of IL-6 production by astaxanthin via ERK-, MSK-, and NF-κB-mediated signals in activated microglia." *International immunopharmacology* 10.12 (2010): 1560-1572.

11. Xu, Lianbao, et al. "Astaxanthin improves cognitive deficits from oxidative stress, nitric oxide synthase and inflammation through upregulation of PI3K/ Akt in diabetes rat." *International journal of clinical and experimental pathology* 8.6 (2015): 6083.

12. Zhang, Xiang-Sheng, et al. "Astaxanthin offers neuroprotection and reduces neuroinflammation in experimental subarachnoid hemorrhage." *journal of surgical research* 192.1 (2014): 206-213.

13. Zhou, Liping, et al. "Protective effect of astaxanthin against multiple organ injury in a rat model of sepsis." *journal of surgical research* 195.2 (2015): 559-567.

14. Baralic, Ivana, et al. "Effect of astaxanthin supplementation on salivary IgA, oxidative stress, and inflammation in young soccer players." *Evidence-Based Complementary and Alternative Medicine* 2015 (2015).

15. Park, J. S., et al. "Astaxanthin modulates age-associated mitochondrial dysfunction in healthy dogs." *Journal of animal science* 91.1 (2013): 268-275.

16. Yuan and Kijita 2009 in Kidd, Parris. "Astaxanthin, cell membrane nutrient with diverse clinical benefits and anti-aging potential." *Altern Med Rev* 16.4 (2011): 355-64.

17. Piermarocchi, Stefano, et al. "Carotenoids in Age-related Maculopathy Italian Study (CARMIS): two-year results of a randomized study." *European journal of ophthalmology* 22.2 (2012): 216.

18. Lyons, Nicole M., and Nora M. O'Brien. "Modulatory effects of an algal extract containing astaxanthin on UVAirradiated cells in culture." *Journal of dermatological science* 30.1 (2002): 73-84.

19. Tominaga, Kumi, et al. "Cosmetic benefits of astaxanthin on humans subjects." *Acta Biochimica Polonica* 59.1 (2012): 43.

20. Aoi, Wataru, et al. "Astaxanthin limits exercise-induced skeletal and cardiac muscle damage in mice." *Antioxidants and Redox Signaling* 5.1 (2003): 139-144.

21. Polotow, Tatiana G., et al. "Astaxanthin supplementation delays physical exhaustion and prevents redox imbalances in plasma and soleus muscles of Wistar

rats." *Nutrients* 6.12 (2014): 5819-5838.

NAD

1. Trammell, Samuel AJ, et al. "Nicotinamide riboside is a major NAD+ precursor vitamin in cow milk." *The Journal of nutrition* 146.5 (2016): 957-963.

2. Ziegler, Mathias, and Marc Niere. "NAD+ surfaces again." *Biochemical Journal* 382.3 (2004): E5.

3. Denu, John M. "Vitamins and aging: pathways to NAD+ synthesis." *Cell* 129.3 (2007): 453-454.

4. Gomes, Ana P., et al. "Declining NAD+ induces a pseudohypoxic state disrupting nuclear-mitochondrial communication during aging." *Cell* 155.7 (2013): 1624-1638.

5. Mouchiroud, Laurent, Riekelt H. Houtkooper, and Johan Auwerx. "NAD+ metabolism: a therapeutic target for agerelated metabolic disease." *Critical reviews in biochemistry and molecular biology* 48.4 (2013): 397-408.

6. Lin, Su-Ju, and Leonard Guarente. "Nicotinamide adenine dinucleotide, a metabolic regulator of transcription, longevity and disease." *Current opinion in cell biology* 15.2 (2003): 241-246.

7. Stein, Liana Roberts, and Shin-ichiro Imai. "The dynamic regulation of NAD metabolism in mitochondria." *Trends in Endocrinology & Metabolism* 23.9 (2012): 420-428.

8. Imai, Shin-ichiro, and Leonard Guarente. "NAD+ and sirtuins in aging and disease." *Trends in cell biology* 24.8 (2014): 464-471.

9. Zhang, Hongbo, et al. "NAD+ repletion improves mitochondrial and stem cell function and enhances life span in mice." *Science* 352.6292 (2016): 1436-1443.

10. Mendelsohn, Andrew R., and James W. Larrick. "Partial reversal of skeletal muscle aging by restoration of normal NAD+ levels." *Rejuvenation research* 17.1 (2014): 62-69.

11. Sauve, Anthony A. "NAD+ and vitamin B3: from metabolism to therapies." *Journal of pharmacology and experimental therapeutics* 324.3 (2008): 883-893.

12. Brown, Kevin D., et al. "Activation of SIRT3 by the NAD+ precursor nicotinamide riboside protects from noiseinduced hearing loss." *Cell metabolism* 20.6 (2014): 1059-1068.

CURCUMIN

1. Shen, Li-Rong, et al. "Curcumin and aging." *Biofactors* 39.1 (2013): 133-140.

2. Aggarwal, Bharat B., Subash C. Gupta, and Bokyung Sung. "Curcumin: an orally bioavailable blocker of TNF and other pro-inflammatory biomarkers." *British journal of pharmacology* 169.8 (2013): 1672-1692.

3. Barzegar, Abolfazl, and Ali A. Moosavi-Movahedi. "Intracellular ROS protection efficiency and free radicalscavenging activity of curcumin." *PLoS One* 6.10 (2011): e26012.

4. Trujillo, Joyce, et al. "Mitochondria as a target in the therapeutic properties of curcumin." *Archiv der Pharmazie* 347.12 (2014): 873-884.

5. Kim, Teayoun, et al. "Curcumin activates AMPK and suppresses gluconeogenic gene expression in hepatoma cells." *Biochemical and biophysical research communications* 388.2 (2009): 377-382.

6. Xiao, Kui, et al. "Curcumin induces autophagy via activating the AMPK signaling pathway in lung adenocarcinoma cells." *Journal of pharmacological sciences* 123.2 (2013): 102-109.

7. Pu, Yunfei, et al. "Dietary curcumin ameliorates aging-related cerebrovascular dysfunction through the AMPK/ uncoupling protein 2 pathway." *Cellular Physiology and Biochemistry* 32.5 (2013): 1167-1177.

8. Panahi, Yunes, et al. "A randomized controlled trial on the anti-inflammatory effects of curcumin in patients with chronic sulphur mustard-induced cutaneous complications." *Annals of clinical biochemistry* 49.6 (2012): 580-588.

9. Gupta, Subash C., Sridevi Patchva, and Bharat B. Aggarwal. "Therapeutic roles of curcumin: lessons learned from clinical trials." *The AAPS journal* 15.1 (2013): 195-218.

10. Julie, S., and M. T. Jurenka. "Anti-inflammatory properties of curcumin, a major constituent." *Alternative medicine review* 14.2 (2009).

11. Kuptniratsaikul, Vilai, et al. "Efficacy and safety of Curcuma domestica extracts in patients with knee osteoarthritis." *The Journal of Alternative and Complementary Medicine* 15.8 (2009): 891-897.

12. Tang, Youcai, and Anping Chen. "Curcumin eliminates the effect of advanced glycation end-products (AGEs) on the divergent regulation of gene expression of receptors of AGEs by interrupting leptin signaling." *Laboratory Investigation* 94.5 (2014): 503-516.

13. Zorofchian Moghadamtousi, Soheil, et al. "A review on antibacterial, antiviral, and antifungal activity of curcumin." *BioMed research international* 2014 (2014).

14. Rastogi, Manisha, et al. "Protective effect of curcuminoids on age-related mitochondrial impairment in female Wistar rat brain." *Biogerontology* 15.1 (2014): 21-31.

15. Antony, B., et al. "A Pilot Cross-Over Study to Evaluate Human Oral Bioavailability of BCM-95? CG (BiocurcumaxTM), A Novel Bioenhanced Preparation of Curcumin." *Indian journal of pharmaceutical sciences* 70.4 (2008): 445.

CARNOSINE

1. Barron, J. 2012. "Carnosine, still the best for Anti-aging." *Baseline of Health Foundation. Health Newsletter.* 2012.

2. A Babizhayev, Mark, and Yegor E Yegorov. "An "Enigmatic" L-Carnosine (β-Alanyl-L-Histidine)? Cell Proliferative Activity as a Fundamental Property

of a Natural Dipeptide Inherent to Traditional Antioxidant, Anti-Aging Biological Activities: Balancing and a Hormonally Correct Agent, Novel Patented Oral Therapy Dosage Formulation for Mobility, Skeletal Muscle Power and Functional Performance, Hypothalamic-Pituitary-Brain Relationship in Health, Aging and Stress Studies." *Recent patents on drug delivery & formulation* 9.1 (2015): 1-64.

3. Boldyrev, Alexander A., Giancarlo Aldini, and Wim Derave. "Physiology and pathophysiology of carnosine." *Physiological reviews* 93.4 (2013): 1803-1845.

4. Budzeń, Sandra, and Joanna Rymaszewska. "The biological role of carnosine and its possible applications in medicine." Advances in clinical and experimental medicine: *official organ Wroclaw Medical University* 22.5 (2012): 739-744.

5. Holliday, Robin, and G. A. McFarland. "Inhibition of the growth of transformed and neoplastic cells by the dipeptide carnosine." *British journal of cancer* 73.8 (1996): 966.

6. Hipkiss, Alan R., Estifanos Baye, and Barbora de Courten. "Carnosine and the processes of ageing." *Maturitas* 93 (2016): 28-33.

7. Kyriazis, Marios. *Carnosine and Other Elixirs of Youth: The Miraculous Anti-ageing Supplement.* Watkins, 2003.

8. Wang, A. M., et al. "Use of carnosine as a natural anti-senescence drug for human beings." *Biochemistry C/C of Biokhimiia*

65.7 (2000): 869-871.

9. Park, Hui-Seung, et al. "The neuroprotective effects of carnosine in early stage of focal ischemia rodent model." *Journal of Korean Neurosurgical Society* 55.3 (2014): 125-130.

10. Prokopieva, V. D., et al. "Use of carnosine for oxidative stress reduction in different pathologies." *Oxidative medicine and cellular longevity* 2016 (2016).

11. Yan, Hong, et al. "Effect of carnosine, aminoguanidine, and aspirin drops on the prevention of cataracts in diabetic rats." (2008).

12. Song, Byeng Chun, et al. "Biological functions of histidine-dipeptides and metabolic syndrome." *Nutrition research and practice* 8.1 (2014): 3-10.

13. Shao, Lan, Qing-huan Li, and Zheng Tan. "L-carnosine reduces telomere damage and shortening rate in cultured normal fibroblasts." *Biochemical and biophysical research communications* 324.2 (2004): 931-936.

14. Hipkiss, Alan R. "Possible benefit of dietary carnosine towards depressive disorders." *Aging and disease* 6.5 (2015): 300.

15. Cararo, J. H., Streck, E. L., Schuck, P. F., & da C Ferreira, G. (2015). Carnosine and related peptides: Therapeutic potential in age-related disorders. *Aging and disease,* 6(5), 369.

16. Maes, D. Cited in Harpers Bazaar (British ed.) Nov 2007

17. Babizhayev, Mark A., et al.

"N-Acetylcarnosine sustained drug delivery eye drops to control the signs of ageless vision: Glare sensitivity, cataract amelioration and quality of vision currently available treatment for the challenging 50,000-patient population." *Clin Interv Aging* 4.1 (2009): 31-50.

18. Babizhayev, Mark A., et al. "N-acetylcarnosine lubricant eyedrops possess all-in-one universal antioxidant protective effects of L-carnosine in aqueous and lipid membrane environments, aldehyde scavenging, and transglycation activities inherent to cataracts: a clinical study of the new vision-saving drug N-acetylcarnosine eyedrop therapy in a database population of over 50,500 patients." *American journal of therapeutics* 16.6 (2009): 517-533.

19. Babizhayev, Mark A., and Anatoly I. Deyev. "Management of the virulent influenza virus infection by oral formulation of nonhydrolized carnosine and isopeptide of carnosine attenuating proinflammatory cytokine-induced nitric oxide production." *American journal of therapeutics* 19.1 (2012): e25-e47.

20. Sale, Craig, et al. "Carnosine: from exercise performance to health." *Amino Acids* 44.6 (2013): 1477-1491.

METFORMIN

1. Haiken, M. "Common Drug Has the Potential to slow Aging, Boost Cancer Recovery." *In Forbes Mag.* March. 2013

2. Anisimov, Vladimir N. "Metformin:

do we finally have an anti-aging drug?." *Cell Cycle* 12.22 (2013): 3483-3489.

3. Bannister, CA 1., et al. "Can people with type 2 diabetes live longer than those without? A comparison of mortality in people initiated with metformin or sulphonylurea monotherapy and matched, non-diabetic controls." *Diabetes, Obesity and Metabolism* 16.11 (2014): 1165-1173.

4. Na, Hyun-Jin, et al. "Mechanism of metformin: Inhibition of DNA damage and proliferative activity in Drosophila midgut stem cell." *Mechanisms of ageing and development* 134.9 (2013): 381-390.

5. Lee, Yong-Syu, et al. "Combined metformin and resveratrol confers protection against UVC-induced DNA damage in A549 lung cancer cells via modulation of cell cycle checkpoints and DNA repair." *Oncology reports* 35.6 (2016): 3735-3741.

6. Zhong, T., et al. "Metformin alters DNA methylation genome-wide via the H19/SAHH axis." Oncogene (2016).

7. Martin-Montalvo, Alejandro, et al. "Metformin improves healthspan and lifespan in mice." *Nature communications* 4 (2013).

8. Viollet, Benoit, et al. "Cellular and molecular mechanisms of metformin: an overview." *Clinical science* 122.6 (2012): 253-270.

9. Pryor, Rosina, and Filipe Cabreiro. "Repurposing metformin: an old drug with new tricks in its binding pockets." *Biochemical Journal*

471.3 (2015): 307-322.

10. Hattori, Yuichi, Kohshi Hattori, and Toshio Hayashi. "Pleiotropic benefits of metformin: macrophage targeting its anti-inflammatory mechanisms." *Diabetes* 64.6 (2015): 1907-1909.

11. Fatt, Michael, et al. "Metformin acts on two different molecular pathways to enhance adult neural precursor proliferation/self-renewal and differentiation." *Stem cell reports* 5.6 (2015): 988-995.

12. Na, Hyun-Jin, et al. "Mechanism of metformin: Inhibition of DNA damage and proliferative activity in Drosophila midgut stem cell." *Mechanisms of ageing and development* 134.9 (2013): 381-390.

13. Blagosklonny, Mikhail V. "Why men age faster but reproduce longer than women: mTOR and evolutionary perspectives." *Aging (Albany NY)* 2.5 (2010): 265-273.

14. Badr, D., M. Kurban, and O. Abbas. "Metformin in dermatology: an overview." *Journal of the European Academy of Dermatology and Venereology* 27.11 (2013): 1329-1335.

ALPHA LIPOIC ACID

1. Shay, Kate Petersen, et al. "Alpha-lipoic acid as a dietary supplement: molecular mechanisms and therapeutic potential." *Biochimica et Biophysica Acta (BBA)-General Subjects* 1790.10 (2009): 1149-1160.

2. Wood, Shona H., et al. "Transcriptome analysis in calorie-restricted rats implicates epigenetic and post-translational mechanisms

in neuroprotection and aging." *Genome biology* 16.1 (2015): 285.

3. Xiong, Shiqin, et al. "PGC-1α modulates telomere function and DNA damage in protecting against aging-related chronic diseases." *Cell reports* 12.9 (2015): 1391-1399.

4. Mendelsohn, Andrew R., and James W. Larrick. "Telomerase reverse transcriptase and peroxisome proliferatoractivated receptor γ co-activator-1α cooperate to protect cells from DNA damage and mitochondrial dysfunction in vascular senescence." *Rejuvenation research* 18.5 (2015): 479-483.

5. Gorąca, Anna, et al. "Lipoic acid–biological activity and therapeutic potential." *Pharmacological Reports* 63.4 (2011): 849-858.

6. Laher, Issy. "Diabetes and alpha lipoic acid." *Frontiers in pharmacology* 2 (2011): 69.

7. Packer, Lester, and Enrique Cadenas. "Lipoic acid: energy metabolism and redox regulation of transcription and cell signaling." *Journal of clinical biochemistry and nutrition* 48.1 (2010): 26-32.

8. Jiang, Tianyi, et al. "Lipoic acid restores age-associated impairment of brain energy metabolism through the modulation of Akt/JNK signaling and PGC1α transcriptional pathway." *Aging cell* 12.6 (2013): 1021-1031.

9. Nebbioso, Marcella, et al. "Biomolecular modulation of neurodegenerative events during ageing." *Oxidative medicine and cellular longevity* 2015 (2015).

10. Gomes, Marilia Brito, and Carlos

Antonio Negrato. "Alpha-lipoic acid as a pleiotropic compound with potential therapeutic use in diabetes and other chronic diseases." *Diabetology & metabolic syndrome* 6.1 (2014): 80.

11. Mahmoud, Y. I., and H. G. Hegazy. "Ginger and alpha lipoic acid ameliorate age-related ultrastructural changes in rat liver." *Biotechnic & Histochemistry* 91.2 (2016): 86-95.

12. Vallianou, Natalia, Angelos Evangelopoulos, and Pavlos Koutalas. "Alpha-lipoic acid and diabetic neuropathy." *Rev Diabet Stud* 6.4 (2009): 230-236.

APIGENIN

1. Paredes-Gonzalez, Ximena, et al. "Apigenin reactivates Nrf2 anti-oxidative stress signaling in mouse skin epidermal JB6 P+ cells through epigenetics modifications." *The AAPS journal* 16.4 (2014): 727-735.

2. Escande, Carlos, et al. "Flavonoid Apigenin Is an Inhibitor of the NAD+ ase CD38." *Diabetes* 62.4 (2013): 1084-1093.

3. Zhang, Y., et al. "Apigenin induces dermal collagen synthesis via smad2/3 signaling pathway." European Journal of Histochemistry 59.2 (2015).

4. Feng, X., et al. "Activation of PPARg by a Natural Flavonoid Modulator, Apigenin Ameliorates Obesity- Related Inflammation Via Regulation of Macrophage Polarization." *EBioMedicine* 9 (2016): 61-76.

5. Wang, Jia, et al. "Apigenin inhibits the expression of IL-6, IL-8, and ICAM-1 in DEHP-stimulated

human umbilical vein endothelial cells and in vivo." *Inflammation* 35.4 (2012): 1466-1476.

6. Lim, Ratana, et al. "Dietary phytophenols curcumin, naringenin and apigenin reduce infection-induced inflammatory and contractile pathways in human placenta, foetal membranes and myometrium." *Molecular human reproduction* 19.7 (2013): 451-462.

7. Choi, S. et al. "Apigenin inhibits UVA-induced cytotoxicity in vitro and prevents signs of aging in vivo." *Internal Journal of Molecular Medicine.* 38; 627-634.(2016)

SULFORAPHANE

1. Zanichelli, Fulvia, et al. "Dose-dependent effects of R-sulforaphane isothiocyanate on the biology of human mesenchymal stem cells, at dietary amounts, it promotes cell proliferation and reduces senescence and apoptosis, while at anti-cancer drug doses, it has a cytotoxic effect." *Age* 34.2 (2012): 281-293.

2. Kaufman-Szymczyk, Agnieszka, et al. "The role of sulforaphane in epigenetic mechanisms, including interdependence between histone modification and DNA methylation." *International journal of molecular sciences* 16.12 (2015): 29732-29743.

3. Dias, Irundika HK, et al. "Sulforaphane restores cellular glutathione levels and reduces chronic periodontitis neutrophil hyperactivity in vitro." *PLoS One* 8.6 (2013): e66407.

4. Houghton, Christine A., Robert G. Fassett, and Jeff S. Coombes.

"Sulforaphane and other nutrigenomic Nrf2 activators: can the clinician's expectation be matched by the reality?." *Oxidative medicine and cellular longevity* 2016 (2016).

5. O'Mealey, Gary B., William L. Berry, and Scott M. Plafker. "Sulforaphane is a Nrf2-independent inhibitor of mitochondrial fission." *Redox Biology* 11 (2017): 103-110.

QUERCETIN

1. Nisha, V. M., et al. "Apigenin and quercetin ameliorate mitochondrial alterations by tunicamycin-induced ER stress in 3T3-L1 adipocytes." *Applied biochemistry and biotechnology* 174.4 (2014): 1365-1375.

2. Fürst, Robert, and Ilse Zündorf. "Plant-derived anti-inflammatory compounds: hopes and disappointments regarding the translation of preclinical knowledge into clinical progress." *Mediators of inflammation* 2014 (2014).

3. Ishizawa, Keisuke, et al. "Metabolism of quercetin in vivo and its protective effect against arteriosclerosis." *Journal of Pharmacological Sciences.* Vol. 112. Editorial Off, Kantohya Bldg Gokomachi-Ebisugawa Nakagyo-Ku, Kyoto, 604, Japan: Japanese Pharmacological Soc, 2010.

4. Larson, Abigail J., J. David Symons, and Thunder Jalili. "Therapeutic potential of quercetin to decrease blood pressure: review of efficacy and mechanisms." *Advances in Nutrition: An International Review Journal* 3.1 (2012): 39-46.

5. Costa, Lucio G., et al. "Mechanisms of neuroprotection by quercetin: counteracting oxidative stress and more." *Oxidative medicine and cellular longevity* 2016 (2016).

6. Mlcek, Jiri, et al. "Quercetin and its anti-allergic immune response." *Molecules* 21.5 (2016): 623.

7. Miles, Sarah L., Margaret McFarland, and Richard M. Niles. "Molecular and physiological actions of quercetin: need for clinical trials to assess its benefits in human disease." *Nutrition reviews* 72.11 (2014): 720-734.

8. Hwang, Jin-Taek, Dae Young Kwon, and Suk Hoo Yoon. "AMP-activated protein kinase: a potential target for the diseases prevention by natural occurring polyphenols." *New biotechnology* 26.1 (2009): 17-22.

9. Ahn, Jiyun, et al. "The anti-obesity effect of quercetin is mediated by the AMPK and MAPK signaling pathways." *Biochemical and biophysical research communications* 373.4 (2008): 545-549.

10. Zhu, Yi, et al. "The Achilles' heel of senescent cells: from transcriptome to senolytic drugs." *Aging* cell 14.4 (2015): 644-658.

11. Cherniack, E. Paul. "The potential influence of plant polyphenols on the aging process." *Forschende Komplementärmedizin/Research in Complementary Medicine* 17.4 (2010): 181-187.

EGCG

1. Suzuki, Takuji, et al. "Beneficial Effects of Tea and the Green Tea

Catechin Epigallocatechin-3-gallate on Obesity." *Molecules* 21.10 (2016): 1305.

2. Shin, Joo-Hyun, et al. "Epigallocatechin-3-gallate prevents oxidative stress-induced cellular senescence in human mesenchymal stem cells via Nrf2." *International Journal of Molecular Medicine* 38.4 (2016): 1075-1082.

3. Fürst, Robert, and Ilse Zündorf. "Plant-derived anti-inflammatory compounds: hopes and disappointments regarding the translation of preclinical knowledge into clinical progress." *Mediators of inflammation* 2014 (2014).

4. Singh, Neha Atulkumar, Abul Kalam Azad Mandal, and Zaved Ahmed Khan. "Potential neuroprotective properties of epigallocatechin-3-gallate (EGCG)." *Nutrition journal* 15.1 (2016): 60.

5. Niu, Yucun, et al. "The phytochemical, EGCG, extends lifespan by reducing liver and kidney function damage and improving age-associated inflammation and oxidative stress in healthy rats." *Aging Cell* 12.6 (2013): 1041-1049.

6. Saha, Kamalika, Thomas J. Hornyak, and Richard L. Eckert. "Epigenetic cancer prevention mechanisms in skin cancer." *The AAPS journal* 15.4 (2013): 1064-1071.

7. Martinez-Lopez, Nuria, Diana Athonvarangkul, and Rajat Singh. "Autophagy and aging." *Longevity Genes.* Springer New York, 2015. 73-87.

8. Hwang, Jin-Taek, Dae Young Kwon, and Suk Hoo Yoon. "AMP-activated protein kinase: a potential target for the diseases prevention by natural occurring polyphenols." *New biotechnology* 26.1 (2009): 17-22.

9. Collins, Qu Fan, et al. "Epigallocatechin-3-gallate (EGCG), a green tea polyphenol, suppresses hepatic gluconeogenesis through 5'-AMP-activated protein kinase." *Journal of Biological Chemistry* 282.41 (2007): 30143-30149.

10. Zhou, Jin, et al. "Epigallocatechin-3-gallate (EGCG), a green tea polyphenol, stimulates hepatic autophagy and lipid clearance." *PloS one* 9.1 (2014): e87161.

11. Lagha, Amel Ben, and Daniel Grenier. "Tea polyphenols inhibit the activation of NF-κB and the secretion of cytokines and matrix metalloproteinases by macrophages stimulated with Fusobacterium nucleatum." *Scientific reports* 6 (2016).

12. Oz, Helieh S. "Chronic Inflammatory Diseases and Green Tea Polyphenols." *Nutrients* 9.6 (2017): 561.

13. Sampath, Chethan, et al. "Green tea epigallocatechin 3-gallate alleviates hyperglycemia and reduces advanced glycation end products via nrf2 pathway in mice with high fat diet-induced obesity." *Biomedicine & Pharmacotherapy* 87 (2017): 73-81.

14. Jin, Pan, et al. "Epigallocatechin-3-gallate (EGCG) as a pro-osteogenic agent to enhance osteogenic

differentiation of mesenchymal stem cells from human bone marrow: an in vitro study." *Cell and tissue research* 356.2 (2014): 381-390.

15. Wang, Yanyan, et al. "Green tea epigallocatechin-3-gallate (EGCG) promotes neural progenitor cell proliferation and sonic hedgehog pathway activation during adult hippocampal neurogenesis." *Molecular nutrition & food research* 56.8 (2012): 1292-1303.

ASTRAGALUS

1. Fu, Juan, et al. "Review of the botanical characteristics, phytochemistry, and pharmacology of Astragalus membranaceus (Huangqi)." *Phytotherarearch* 28.9 (2014): 1275-1283.

2. de Jesus, Bruno Bernardes, et al. "The telomerase activator TA-65 elongates short telomeres and increases health span of adult/old mice without increasing cancer incidence." *Aging cell* 10.4 (2011): 604-621.

3. Ip, Fanny CF, et al. "Cycloastragenol is a potent telomerase activator in neuronal cells: implications for depression management." *Neurosignals* 22.1 (2014): 52-63.

4. Reichert, Sophie, et al. "Experimental increase in telomere length leads to faster feather regeneration." *Experimental gerontology* 52 (2014): 36-38.

5. Fauce, Steven Russell, et al. "Telomerase-based pharmacologic enhancement of antiviral function of human CD8+ T lymphocytes." *The Journal of Immunology* 181.10 (2008): 7400-7406.

6. Salvador, Laura, et al. "A natural product telomerase activator lengthens telomeres in humans: a randomized, double blind, and placebo controlled study." *Rejuvenation research* 19.6 (2016): 478-484.

7. Dow, Coad Thomas, and Calvin B. Harley. "Evaluation of an oral telomerase activator for early age-related macular degeneration-a pilot study." *Clinical ophthalmology* (Auckland, NZ) 10 (2016): 243.

8. Sevimli-Gür, Canan, et al. "In vitro growth stimulatory and in vivo wound healing studies on cycloartane-type saponins of Astragalus genus." *Journal of ethnopharmacology* 134.3 (2011): 844-850.

9. Hassan, Samira, Miles Tweed, and Zuchra Zakirova. "Identification of Telomerase-activating Blends From Naturally Occurring Compounds." *Alternative Therapies in Health and Medicine* 22 (2016): 6.

10. Zhang, Xiaohong, and Jiajun Chen. "The mechanism of astragaloside IV promoting sciatic nerve regeneration." *Neural regeneration research* 8.24 (2013): 2256.

11. Jing, Z. H. U., et al. "In vitro intestinal absorption and first-pass intestinal and hepatic metabolism of cycloastragenol, a potent small molecule telomerase activator." *Drug metabolism and pharmacokinetics* 25.5 (2010): 477-486.

MELATONIN

1. Manchester, Lucien C., et al. "Melatonin: an ancient molecule that makes oxygen metabolically tolerable." *Journal of pineal research* 59.4 (2015): 403-419.

2. Jenwitheesuk, Anorut, et al. "Melatonin regulates aging and neurodegeneration through energy metabolism, epigenetics, autophagy and circadian rhythm pathways." *International journal of molecular sciences* 15.9 (2014): 16848-16884.

3. Hardeland, Rüdiger. "Melatonin and the theories of aging: a critical appraisal of melatonin's role in anti-aging mechanisms." *Journal of pineal research* 55.4 (2013): 325-356.

4. Cano Barquilla, Pilar, et al. "Melatonin normalizes clinical and biochemical parameters of mild inflammation in dietinduced metabolic syndrome in rats." *Journal of pineal research* 57.3 (2014): 280-290.

5. Liu, Jie, Fang Huang, and Hong-Wen He. "Melatonin effects on hard tissues: bone and tooth." *International journal of molecular sciences* 14.5 (2013): 10063-10074.

6. Fischer, Tobias W., et al. "Melatonin enhances antioxidative enzyme gene expression (CAT, GPx, SOD), prevents their UVR-induced depletion, and protects against the formation of DNA damage (8-hydroxy-2'-deoxyguanosine) in ex vivo human skin." *Journal of pineal research* 54.3 (2013): 303-312.

7. Borges, Leandro da Silva, et al. "Melatonin decreases muscular oxidative stress and inflammation induced by strenuous exercise and stimulates growth factor synthesis." *Journal of pineal research* 58.2 (2015): 166-172.

8. Gao, Wenjie, et al. "Melatonin enhances chondrogenic differentiation of human mesenchymal stem cells." *Journal of pineal research* 56.1 (2014): 62-70.

9. Mendes, Caroline, et al. "Adaptations of the aging animal to exercise: role of daily supplementation with melatonin." *Journal of pineal research* 55.3 (2013): 229-239.

10. Pandi-Perumal, Seithikurippu R., et al. "Melatonin antioxidative defense: therapeutical implications for aging and neurodegenerative processes." *Neurotoxicity research* 23.3 (2013): 267-300.

11. Ali, Tahir, et al. "Melatonin attenuates D-galactose-induced memory impairment, neuroinflammation and neurodegeneration via RAGE/NF-KB/JNK signaling pathway in aging mouse model." *Journal of pineal research* 58.1 (2015): 71-85.

12. Calvo-Guirado, José L., et al. "Melatonin stimulates the growth of new bone around implants in the tibia of rabbits." *Journal of pineal research* 49.4 (2010): 356-363.

13. Bejarano, Ignacio, et al. "Exogenous melatonin supplementation prevents oxidative stress-evoked DNA damage in human spermatozoa." *Journal of pineal research* 57.3 (2014): 333-339.

PYRIDOXAMINE

1. Chen, Joline LT, and Jean Francis. "Pyridoxamine, advanced glycation inhibition, and diabetic nephropathy." *Journal of the American Society of Nephrology* 23.1 (2012): 6-8.

2. Voziyan, P. A., and B. G. Hudson. "Pyridoxamine as a multifunctional pharmaceutical: targeting pathogenic glycation and oxidative damage." *Cellular and Molecular Life Sciences* 62.15 (2005): 1671-1681.

3. Chang, Kuo-Chu, et al. "Prevention of arterial stiffening by pyridoxamine in diabetes is associated with inhibition of the pathogenic glycation on aortic collagen." *British journal of pharmacology* 157.8 (2009): 1419-1426.

4. Elseweidy, Mohamed M., et al. "Pyridoxamine, an inhibitor of protein glycation, in relation to microalbuminuria and proinflammatory cytokines in experimental diabetic nephropathy." *Experimental Biology and Medicine* 238.8 (2013): 881-888.

5. Illien-Junger, Svenja, et al. "Combined anti-inflammatory and anti-AGE drug treatments have a protective effect on intervertebral discs in mice with diabetes." *PLoS One* 8.5 (2013): e64302.

Made in the USA
Columbia, SC
09 February 2022